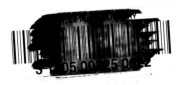

T3-BHM-758

Scoliosis Surgery

The Definitive Patient's Reference

Second Edition

David K. Wolpert

Swordfish Communications, LLC
Austin, Texas

Published by:
Swordfish Communications, LLC
6602 Jamaica Court
Austin, TX 78757 U.S.A.
Fax: (484) 492-7299
www.SwordfishCommunications.com
orders@SwordfishCommunications.com

ISBN-13: 978-0-9741955-1-3
ISBN-10: 0-9741955-1-0

Library of Congress Control Number: 2005903514

Second edition, first printing—May, 2005

Printed in the United States of America

IMPORTANT

The information contained in this book is solely for educational purposes and is not intended as, nor should be considered, medical advice. The ideas, procedures, and suggestions contained in this book are not intended as a substitute for consulting with your physician. Only your physician can provide specific diagnoses and treatments. The author is not responsible for any loss, injury, or damage arising from any use of the information in this book.

Acknowledgements

This book would not have been possible without the generous assistance of many individuals: Mary Albertson; Kevin C. Booth, M.D.; Jeffrey Bratberg, PharmD, BCPS; Steven Bratberg; Lisa Cowger; Tracy Gaudu, P.A.; Tiffany Ann Jackson; Michael O. LaGrone, M.D.; John P. Lubicky, M.D.; Beth McHugh; Cheryl Klinginsmith; Don Perkins; Linda Racine; Trent Reynolds; Travis Roper; Janice and Stanley Sacks; Cindy Savage; and Kurt W. Von Rueden, M.D.

I would also like to thank my family and friends for their ongoing support, encouragement, and advice as I recovered from surgery and became inspired to write this book.

Finally, I must thank all of those with scoliosis and their families who shared their stories with me and provided invaluable feedback on the first edition. This book is for you.

— *David Wolpert*

Contents

Preface

This is the book I wish I had read before I had scoliosis surgery. Despite my enormous respect for surgeons, they are often not the best communicators for those who want explanations in simple terms, or for those who want the brutally honest truth without all the qualifiers medical professionals frequently put on unpleasant news. As a result, many patients turn to support groups, Internet discussion boards, or other places for answers. Some people will find the answers they need there. Others will be bewildered by the overwhelming amount of inaccuracy and confusion about scoliosis. Trying to ascertain what is correct or relevant and what is not is tedious, frustrating, and often impossible. I looked for a single book, a paper, a website, or *anything* that could answer all my questions about scoliosis surgery, thoroughly and honestly. I could not find one, so I decided to write my own.

My goal was to write a book that would explain everything you need to know to help you make the decision whether to have surgery, how to prepare for it if you decide to proceed, and how to cope with the lengthy recovery process. I thought it was critical that the book be written in plain English while simultaneously giving you the tools to understand the medical jargon you will surely encounter. The information in this book is based on published research, interviews with orthopedic surgeons, discussions with people who have been through the surgery, and my own experience.

This book is not for everyone. I focus exclusively on scoliosis surgery and therefore do not address topics such as bracing as a treatment for adolescents, the importance of early detection, or research into the possible causes of the disorder. In addition, this is a very to-the-point book. Unlike other books on scoliosis, I do not include dozens of personal stories because I feel they detract from the key points you need to know. Finally, this book is perfectly applicable to people of all ages who are facing scoliosis surgery, but it is written for a more mature reader. Appendix B lists some good books for those who want to know more about the things not included here, and for younger readers.

It would be irresponsible of me to suggest that this book is truly all you need to know. Every scoliosis case is different. This book cannot replace the advice of your orthopedist, and you should not take anything in this book as medical advice.

I sincerely hope this book helps you make the decisions that are right *for you.*

My best wishes,
David Wolpert

Scoliosis Surgery

The Definitive Patient's Reference

CHAPTER ONE

Scoliosis Demystified

This chapter will provide you with a sound understanding of scoliosis, commonly referred to as "curvature of the spine." The concepts and terms introduced here are key to understanding the rest of this book. This information will also enable you to speak and understand the language your orthopedic surgeon and other medical providers will use when discussing your case with you.

The Normal Spine

Before discussing scoliosis, it is useful first to understand the anatomy of a normal spine. The spine has four major components: twenty-four individual bones called *vertebrae*, the *sacrum*, the *coccyx*, and *intervertebral discs*.

The set of vertebrae are divided into three groups: the *cervical*, *thoracic*, and *lumbar* regions (Figure 1). The spine consists of seven cervical, twelve thoracic, and five lumbar vertebrae. Spine surgeons refer to each vertebra as a *segment*, or *level*. Each segment can be uniquely identified by a combination of a letter (C, T, or L, for cervical, thoracic, and lumbar, respectively) followed by a number that represents the vertebra's position from the top of a particular region. For example, the fourth vertebra from the top of the thoracic region is called T4.

As shown in Figure 2, each vertebra in the spinal column consists of the vertebral body in the front, two facet joints in the back, and the pedicles, which join the vertebral bodies to the facet joints. The facet joints connect vertebrae together. Between the vertebral bodies are *intervertebral discs* (commonly just called *discs*). These discs allow you to bend and twist, and they cushion impacts to the spine as you run, jump, or exert other forces on your body. The surface of a disc is rough and fibrous, while its inside is soft, with a gel-like texture.

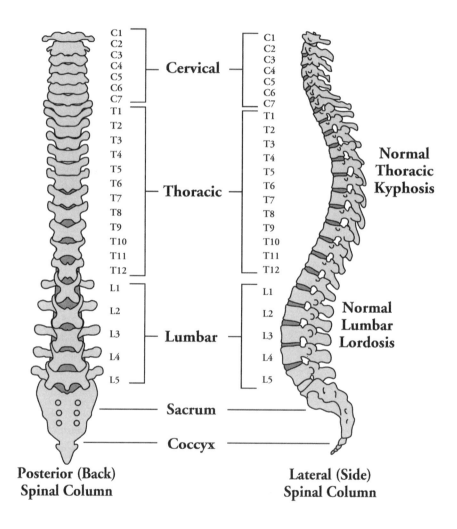

Figure 1: Regions of the spine and sagittal curves

At the lower end of the spine are two other bones: the triangular-shaped *sacrum* and, just below it, the *coccyx*, or tailbone. At birth, your sacrum comprises five distinct bones that fuse together naturally as you grow. These are designated S1 through S5, though this distinction is not really important. The coccyx consists of three small bones, which have no special designation.

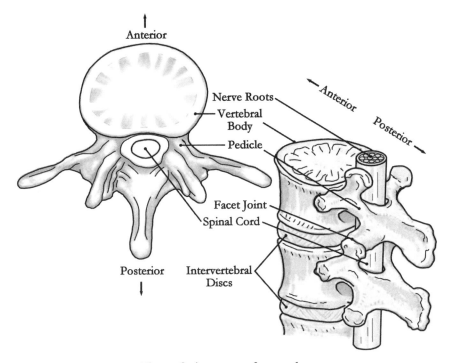

Figure 2: Anatomy of a vertebra

A normal spine is not straight in all dimensions. Viewed from behind, a normal spine is straight *laterally* (from side-to-side). Viewed from the side, however, the normal spine curves slightly inward in the lower back (the lumbar region) and curves slightly outward in the middle back (the thoracic region). These natural bends are called the *sagittal curves*. The inward lumbar curve is called *lordosis*, while the outward thoracic curve is called *kyphosis*.

You may have heard of people having the *condition* of kyphosis or lordosis. The terminology here is confusing. People with *too much* of a kyphotic curvature are said to have *abnormal kyphosis*, which is more commonly called *hunchback* or *roundback*. People with *too little* lumbar lordosis are said to have *abnormal lumbar lordosis*, which, if the loss is severe, is commonly called *flatback* or *flatback syndrome*. It is possible to have either of these conditions in addition to scoliosis.

Defining Scoliosis

The term "scoliosis" is derived from an ancient Greek word meaning "crookedness." In modern parlance, scoliosis is a disorder (not a disease) that describes a curvature of the spine. There are two different abnormal curves in most scoliotic patients: a side-to-side, or *lateral* curvature (as opposed to a front-to-back curvature), and a *rotation* of the vertebrae.

Many scoliosis patients have more than one lateral curve. Slight lateral curvatures are not uncommon in the general population and may not warrant concern; the medical community generally considers only curves that exceed 10° in curvature to be scoliotic (the way curves are measured is explained later in this chapter). The lateral curvature alone can negatively affect your appearance. You might, for example, look as if you are persistently bending or slouching to one side.

However, the rotation is often of more concern than the lateral curve, because high degrees of rotation in the thoracic region pose health risks in addition to cosmetic concerns. As a lateral curve *progresses*, or increases in severity with growth or over time, the amount of rotation also increases. The rotation of the thoracic vertebrae causes the rib cage to rotate, thus compressing the heart and lungs, which are contained within the rib cage. This compression can cause serious heart or breathing problems. Thoracic rotation also induces a more drastic appearance issue—a protruding shoulder blade area called a *rib hump*. Because it is important to treat both of these curves, a more precise definition of scoliosis is a lateral spinal curvature of at least 10° that is usually (though not always) accompanied by a rotation of the vertebrae.

The mechanics of scoliosis are not well understood. The initial cause of most cases of scoliosis is unknown. What is known is that as curvatures increase, the vertebrae involved in the curve begin to change. Bone is living tissue that can deform in response to the lateral imbalance of a scoliotic spine. Over time, the unequal loads placed on either side of a scoliotic spine can cause the shape of certain vertebra to malform, and the discs and facet joints to degenerate unevenly. These are reactionary changes, not causal factors. What initiates the imbalance in the first place is a mystery.

Causes of Scoliosis

It is difficult for many people with scoliosis to accept, but the truth is that nobody knows what causes the majority of scoliosis cases. 75-85% of scoliosis cases are *idiopathic*, meaning *of unknown cause*. As you research scoliosis, you may encounter dozens of theories on what causes scoliosis, such as vitamin deficiencies or lack of certain sugars. Most of these theories are unfounded and should be ignored. It *is* known that there is a genetic basis to scoliosis, evidenced by the fact that scoliosis tends to run in families. Someday, advances in genetic engineering may be able to repair whatever genetic errors pre-disposes one to scoliosis, but for now you need to accept your situation and seek appropriate treatment. You should also accept that there is nothing you could have done to prevent the onset of scoliosis. It is not, as some speculate, caused by behaviors such as maintaining poor posture or carrying heavy bags. It is not your or your parents' fault.

15-25% of scoliosis cases are a byproduct of other known conditions. These include neuromuscular disorders (cerebral palsy, spina bifida, muscular dystrophy, etc.), connective tissue disorders (Marfan Syndrome), and genetic abnormalities (Down Syndrome). In some of these conditions, the muscles or nerves around the spine do not function correctly and cannot support the spine in a straight position. In addition, a child may be born with a curved spine, a condition called *congenital scoliosis*. In older patients, vertebral disc degeneration and arthritis may also cause scoliosis to develop. The same surgery appropriate for those with idiopathic scoliosis may also be appropriate for those with scoliosis caused by these conditions. However, these cases can be quite complex, and it is beyond the scope of this book to address the differences in treating scoliosis resulting from these disorders.

The types of scoliosis described above are sometimes referred to as *structural scoliosis*—cases in which the spine has some degree of permanent (or *fixed*) curvature. There are also cases of what is known as *nonstructural scoliosis* or *functional scoliosis*. This refers to a spinal curvature caused by things other than genetic triggers or known medical conditions. For example, a severe sports injury may cause muscle spasms or inflammation in the tissues surrounding the spine that can push the spine out of alignment. This kind of scoliosis is usually temporary and is not treated surgically. A difference in the length of one of your legs can also cause nonstructural scoliosis, which is easily remedied with a shoe insert. This book does not address nonstructural scoliosis. Note that nonstructural scoliosis is not the same thing as a nonstructural curve, which is defined in the next section.

Classifying Scoliotic Curves

An orthopedist may have told you that you have "idiopathic scoliosis, with a right thoracic structural curve and a compensatory lumbar curve." This section will help you decode such language so that you can better communicate with your surgeon and focus additional research you may conduct on your specific type of scoliosis.

Cases of scoliosis are typically classified in several dimensions: age of onset, cause, the nature of the curve, and the location, type, and convexity of the curve.

Age of onset. This is the age at which your curvature first developed. It is classified either as congenital (scoliosis that developed due to a birth defect), infantile (from birth to age three), juvenile (ages three to ten), adolescent (ages ten to eighteen, or whenever skeletal maturity is reached), or adult (explained below). Most people with scoliosis developed the condition in their teenage years during their growth spurt.

There are two types of adult scoliosis. The more common type is a scoliotic curve that developed prior to age eighteen but continues to progress even though the patient's bones have finished growing (have reached *skeletal maturity*). This is called *adult idiopathic scoliosis.* The less common type is called *de novo scoliosis,* which is scoliosis that develops later in life, typically after the age of forty. It is believed to be caused by degeneration in the discs and facet joints of the spine and is usually related to arthritis or osteoporosis. It may also be referred to as *degenerative scoliosis.* *De novo* scoliosis typically affects only the lumbar region of the spine.

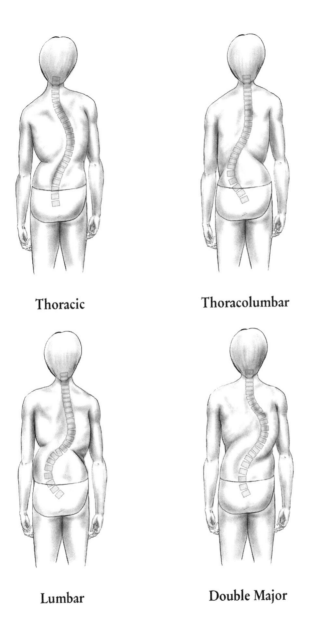

Thoracic   Thoracolumbar

Lumbar   Double Major

Figure 3: Severe cases of the four most common curve types

It is important not to confuse the initial onset of scoliosis with the timing of diagnosis. The latter may postdate the former by many years. It is possible to reach adulthood without ever knowing you have scoliosis, even though it probably developed in your adolescent years.

Cause. As mentioned in the previous section, the cause of most scoliosis cases is unknown (idiopathic) but in some cases a cause can be attributed.

Structural versus nonstructural curves. Most people with scoliosis have more than one lateral curve in their spine. Each curve can be classified as either *structural* (also called *primary* or *major*) or *nonstructural* (usually called *compensatory*, though also called *secondary* or *minor*). Structural curves are the "real" scoliotic curves. They exhibit some degree of permanent curvature because the curve is rigid. They also tend to be the largest curves. To keep the spine as balanced from side-to-side as possible, other sections of the spine may develop a curve in the opposite direction to the structural deformity. These *nonstructural,* or *compensatory,* curves generally remain flexible and are thus not "permanent." *Estimating Correction* (Chapter 2) provides more information on determining the flexibility of curves.

An individual with a right thoracic curve (see below), for example, often has three curves—a structural curve in the thoracic area, and two compensatory curves, one each in the cervical or upper thoracic area and one in the lumbar region. Most surgeons will only operate on the structural curve because the compensatory curves will generally spontaneously realign once the structural curve is reduced. Surgically correcting only the structural section of a curve is called a *selective fusion.*

Note that flexible, nonstructural curves can become progressively more rigid as you age. It is thus possible for a flexible compensatory curve to become a rigid structural curve over time, though this curve would still be considered secondary to the primary curve. It is also possible for a primary curve to be nonstructural, if the scoliosis is caused by a neuromuscular disorder, for example.

Location and convexity of the curve. Over 90% of all scoliotic curves exhibit one of four patterns, which are described below.

It is helpful to be familiar with three terms commonly used to describe curves: convex, concave, and apex. *Convexity* is the direction in which a particular curve bends, or "points" (to the right, or to the left). The convex side of the curve is the outer angle; the concave side is the inner angle. The *apex* of the curve is the most deviated, or off-center, vertebra. If you consider the curve like a mountain, the apex is the peak. There may be more than one apex if you have multiple curves. The most common curve types are:

1. *Single thoracic.* This is by far the most common curve type. The term "single" implies that there is just one structural curve, and in this case it is located in the thoracic region with an apex between T2 and T11. For unknown reasons, 90% of thoracic curves bend to one's right side. This is therefore called a *right thoracic curve* and is said to have *right convexity*. In most cases, a single thoracic curve is accompanied by two compensatory curves, one in the upper thoracic or cervical region and one in the lumbar region.

2. *Thoracolumbar.* This single structural curve spans both the thoracic as well as the lumbar regions of the spine, with an apex at T12 or L1. 80% of thoracolumbar curves bend to one's left side (*left convexity*).

3. *Lumbar.* As the name implies, this is a structural curve that mainly affects the lumbar region of the spine, with an apex between L1 and L4. 70% of lumbar curves have left convexity.

4. *Double major.* A double major curve has two structural curves. This type of curve is sometimes called an *S* curve, whereas a single structural curve is referred to as a *C* curve. 90% of double major curves include a right thoracic curve and a left lumbar curve, a pattern that resembles a backward S.

Measuring Scoliotic Curves

An orthopedist has probably told you that you have a curve of some specific degree measurement, such as a "50° curve." This section explains what that means. The standard measurement of scoliotic curves is called the *Cobb angle,* named after the orthopedic surgeon who created this approach to measurement (the *Cobb method*).

The first step in determining the magnitude of your curvature is to take a *full-length standing P/A x-ray* of your back. "P/A" stands for posterior/anterior, which in this context means from the back to the front of the body. This type of x-ray picture is taken with the patient standing up, with his or her back facing the x-ray machine. The picture spans the entire back, from the top of the neck all the way down to the pelvis. It may also be necessary to take A/P x-rays (anterior/posterior, taken with the patient facing the x-ray machine), although, for females in particular, this presents a higher risk of radiation exposure to breast tissue.

Your orthopedist will study the x-ray to determine the two *end-vertebrae* in your curve—the vertebrae at the upper and lower extremes of your structural curve. Next, two straight lines are hand-drawn on your x-ray film, one at the top of the highest vertebra in the structural curve and one at the bottom of the lowest vertebra in the structural curve (Figure 4). The orthopedist will then draw lines perpendicular to those lines. The perpendicular lines intersect at an angle. The degree measurement of that angle is the magnitude of your curvature. As mentioned previously, many people with scoliosis have more than one curve, each of which may be either structural or compensatory. Your orthopedist will measure all the curves, but structural curves are the most important.

When documenting a Cobb angle, it is important that the orthopedist or radiologist record not only the upper and lower end-vertebrae used for the calculation, but also which method (e.g. the Cobb method) was utilized. The same vertebrae should be used on subsequent occasions to measure curvature, thereby ensuring that future analyses of your curve's progression are valid "apples-to-apples" comparisons. This information is usually found in the *radiographic report*, which is a short summary of the findings written shortly after the x-rays are taken. These reports become part of your *chart* (a file of your medical records from your interactions with a specific doctor) and therefore last far longer than the x-ray films, which are often discarded from medical records after a few years.

Be aware that the Cobb method is not an exact science. It is prone to human error. One possible error is selecting the wrong vertebrae as the end-points for the top and bottom of the structural curve. An orthopedist may also make small errors in drawing straight lines or in using a protractor or other tool to measure the angle, thus resulting in an inaccurate angle estimation. In addition, the structural measurement of your curvature may be slightly off due to factors beyond the control of the orthopedist, such as precisely how straight you were standing when the x-ray was taken, or even muscle fatigue that can slightly increase your curvature temporarily.

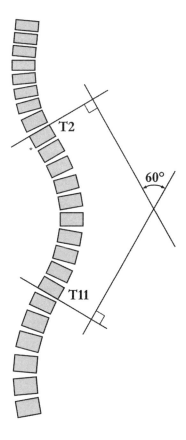

Figure 4: Cobb method measurement example

With these points in mind, you should consider the measurement of your curve to be a good approximation, realizing that the actual curve may vary by a few degrees. According to a study done by the Scoliosis Research Society, differences in measurement by a particular orthopedist of an identical x-ray may vary over time by as much as 5°, while differences in measurement between orthopedists may vary by as much as 10°. The implication of this variance is that you should not be alarmed if your curve measurement increases by a degree or two. Likewise, a slight reduction in curve measurement does not necessarily mean your curvature has actually improved.

0: No rotation. Pedicles equidistant from midline.

+1: Both pedicles visible but not equidistant from midline

+2: One pedicle almost on midline, the other only partially visible

+3: One pedicle on midline, the other not visible

+4: One pedicle beyond midline, the other not visible

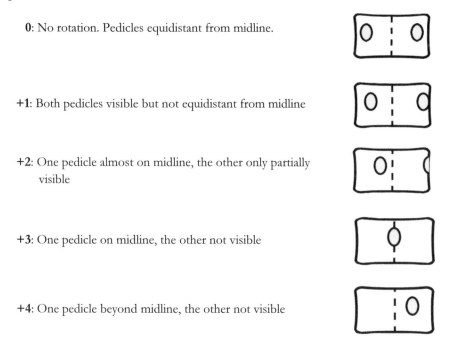

Figure 5: Rotation measurements

In addition to the lateral curvature, the rotation of the spine can also be measured. This is done by observing how far the *pedicles* of the vertebra at the apex of the curve deviate from the *midline*. The pedicles are seen on x-ray films as small oval indentations on either side of the vertebra. The midline is an imaginary vertical line drawn down the middle of a hypothetically straight spine. The two pedicles in a non-rotated vertebra should be equidistant from the midline. An arbitrary scale of 0-4 is used to describe the relative proximity of the pedicles to the midline (Figure 5). The amount of rotation would be reported as something like a "+3 rotation."

Progression is the Enemy

A curved spine, by itself, is not necessarily cause for alarm. Millions of Americans of all ages have a mild curvature (under 20°) and yet experience no problems—they do not look abnormal, they do not have pain, and their flexibility is not noticeably impaired. At the same time, many people have moderate curvatures but, even though they may have some noticeable deformity or pain, do not find that these issues impede their quality of life or degrade their self-image. Scoliosis is not necessarily a problem if the curve is stable and the patient has no significant pain or aesthetic concerns.

However, the situation is more complex if a patient has a documented history of curve progression. The term *progression* simply means "getting worse," specifically, by an increase of 5° or more over successive measurements. Over time, some curves progress while others do not. Why only certain curves progress is not understood. If curves progress beyond a certain threshold, serious complications can arise (see *Risks of Severe or Progressing Curvatures*).

The best predictor of future progression is past progression. The only way to verify that a curve is progressing is to compare its current Cobb angle to levels at which it was previously measured. The time lapse required between measurements varies. Some curves progress as slowly as 1° per year, while in some cases, curves progress so rapidly that it can be quickly determined that a curve is progressing. Curves tend to progress most rapidly during the formative years and, in particular, during the adolescent growth spurt. Increases in curvature of 20-30° per year in a child are not uncommon.

Because Cobb angle measurements are not always consistently accurate with repeated measurement, a curve may need to progress several degrees before it can be classified as progressive. Consider, for example, a curve that progresses 1° per year for five years. Since there is an inherent "plus or minus 5°" margin of error in Cobb angle measurements, it would not be definitive to say that a curve that measures 5° more than it did five years prior is actually progressing. In contrast, ten years of progression at 1° per year would be strong evidence.

Proving the progression of a curvature over time can be difficult if old x-rays are not available. If x-rays of your spine were ever taken—either for scoliosis, perhaps after an accident you had, or for any other reason—the facility where they were taken or evaluated may still have the originals, or copies on microfilm. Records older than approximately seven years are often destroyed or transferred to microfilm and moved to off-site storage facilities. The records department of most medical facilities can usually assist you in locating these. If you cannot get the x-rays, you may still be able to get old radiological reports that summarize the findings of your old x-rays. These may denote a measurement of your scoliotic curve.

For an adolescent without a documented history of progression, statistics can be used to estimate the probability of a curve's progression based on the Cobb angle when first measured and the current age of the patient. Figure 6 summarizes these probabilities. Remember, the probability of progression in any specific case may be higher or lower.

Patients with a demonstrated history of progression into adulthood will almost certainly continue to progress. For example, the chart indicates that the curves of 30% of 16 year olds with a 30-59° curvature will progress. But the probability that the curve of an adult with a 30-59° degree curvature *whose curve has been progressing steadily since adolescence* will continue to progress is actually closer to 100%.

Other factors can help predict the likelihood of curve progression. For example, scoliotic curves in women are up to ten times more likely to progress than those in men. The type of curve is also a factor. Thoracic curves tend to progress more frequently than do lumbar curves, and spines with two structural curves are more likely to progress than those with a single structural curve.

The rate at which curves progress is not always linear, and curves do not necessarily progress for the entire remainder of one's life. This makes it impossible to predict with certainty an individual's curvature at or by a specific age. Again, however, the best predictor of future progression is past progression. It is reasonable to assume that a curve that has progressed 1° per year

for the last ten years will progress approximately 1° per year for the next ten years.

Cobb angle at initial detection	Age 10-12	Age 13-15	Age 16
<19°	25%	10%	0%
20-29°	60%	40%	10%
30-59°	90%	70%	30%
>60°	100%	90%	70%

**Figure 6: Probabilities of progression in adolescent
idiopathic scoliosis, prior to skeletal maturity**
Source: Scoliosis Research Society, 1982

Slow progressions over time may not warrant concern, but you need to consider the long-term outlook. My curve, as an example, progressed slowly but steadily, increasing 13° over a span of sixteen years, from 36° at age fourteen to 49° at age thirty. That averages out to less than 1° per year, which seems trivial. But, if that trend continued until I was seventy years old, my curve would be a more painful and potentially dangerous 82°.

Risks of Severe or Progressing Curvatures

Even if you are not experiencing any problems you deem significant right now, you should be aware of what problems you may encounter if your curve progresses. More advanced cases of scoliosis have four detrimental effects:

Pain. Statistically, people with scoliosis report only a slightly higher incidence of back pain than the general population. Back pain is actually quite common in the general population, especially among older people. But the *severity* of that pain is typically worse in scoliotic patients and is less responsive to conservative treatments such as painkilling drugs. Pain levels in scoliotic patients generally increase both as a function of age and the severity of the curve: the older you are and the more pronounced your curve is, the higher the pain level you will probably experience.

Back pain can be directly caused by a spinal curvature because the muscles around the spine must work extra hard to maintain a relatively straight posture. This can cause muscle tension, soreness, or other types of pain or discomfort. The stress on the spine can also damage the discs and facet joints between vertebrae, causing arthritic pain in the spine (a condition known as *spondylosis*). Some patients also experience pain in their legs or buttocks, which can be caused by a scoliotic curvature that pinches the nerves that extend down to the legs.

Keep in mind that not all pain experienced by individuals with scoliosis is related to their curvatures. Scoliosis patients are just as likely as anyone else to develop other problems that can cause back or leg pain. Some medical professionals may be quick to dismiss your complaints about back pain by looking at your scoliotic curve and saying, "Well, *of course* you have back pain— look at that curvature!" In reality, the cause of your pain could be something as simple as poor sleeping habits, or as complex as a herniated disc or tumor. Or, yes, it could be related to your scoliosis. This is why it is critical, *before* you commit to having surgery, that you ascertain whether any pain you are experiencing is directly attributable to your scoliosis or to some other factor. An orthopedist with expertise in scoliosis can usually determine whether your pain is related to your curvature. He or she may also refer you to other specialists for further analysis. These specialists, such as pain management specialists or physical therapists, may introduce you to pain management techniques that effectively control your pain such that surgery becomes a less viable course of action for you.

Poor appearance. All spinal deformities impact your appearance to some extent. Many people with scoliosis, even those with moderately severe deformities, look normal to the casual observer. On closer inspection, though, most people with scoliosis have one or more of the following appearance issues: one shoulder higher than the other, a protruding shoulder blade area, an uneven waist line, a "hump" on one side of the back when the person bends forward, or a head that does not point straight ahead when relaxed. These deformities can lead to secondary problems in daily life. For instance, sitting in certain types of chairs may be uncomfortable, or clothing may not fit quite right. In addition, the greater your curvature, the less your apparent height will be.

Cardiopulmonary problems. Severe thoracic curvatures may compress the heart and lungs. This is rarely a problem until the curve reaches at least 70° (some surgeons would say this cutoff is closer to 100°) in magnitude, though some reduction in pulmonary function can be seen at as little as 60°. Thoracic curves that exceed about 80° (again, surgeons vary on the precise cut-off) can cause *restrictive lung disease,* which makes it harder to breathe and reduces the amount of oxygen available to your body and, most importantly, to your heart. Incidentally, regardless of the lateral curvature of the thoracic region, a severe thoracic lordosis can be equally or in some cases even more dangerous.

Neurological problems. A severe curvature of the spine can pinch the nerves contained within the spine. This can lead to pain, numbness, or tingling in the back, legs, or buttocks.

Death. In a very small number of adult cases, the restriction a large thoracic curve (about 100° or more) can place on one's heart and lungs can prove fatal. This is caused either directly by heart failure or in conjunction with complications associated with other serious conditions.

Mortality rates are also significantly higher for children whose curvatures have reached 50° before the age of five. A curvature of that magnitude in a growing child impairs the development of normal lungs.

Putting It All Together

The goal of this chapter was to give you sufficient information to be able to understand what scoliosis is, how your particular case might be defined, and briefly touch on some of the effects of the condition. With this information as a baseline, you now have the basic knowledge and vocabulary to understand what scoliosis surgery is all about, which will be discussed in detail in the next chapter.

CHAPTER TWO

Understanding Spinal Fusion

Scoliosis surgery—technically called *spinal fusion with instrumentation*—is major surgery. Like any surgery, spinal fusion has risks, the recovery can be long and painful, and there may be permanent detrimental effects. As with any surgical procedure, you should consider this surgery a last resort for treatment. This chapter examines the conditions under which surgery should be considered and the surgical options available.

Indications and Contraindications for Surgery

Scoliosis surgery is not for everyone. Medical professionals use the term *indications* to describe the factors that make one a candidate for scoliosis surgery; these are listed below. There are also some factors that *exclude* one from being a viable surgical candidate, which medical professionals call *contraindications*. The term "candidate" is important because scoliosis surgery is almost never a life-or-death decision. If an orthopedic surgeon determines that you are a viable candidate for surgery, the decision whether to proceed is *yours* to make. Be clear: scoliosis surgery is a major operative procedure. The decision whether to have the surgery should not be made hastily. You should absolutely get at least one second opinion.

In general, you are a candidate for scoliosis surgery if any of the following three conditions apply:

Your curve currently exceeds 50°. Some orthopedists may select a different cutoff point; perhaps 45°, or even 60°. The cutoff depends on many factors, such as your age, the location and type of curve, history of curve progression, your level of pain, and the state of your sagittal curves. Note that the majority of curves above 50° will progress, regardless of one's age. If you are an adolescent and still growing, a curve in this range is likely to worsen to a point at which pain and serious medical complications may arise, thus making you an excellent candidate for surgery. On the other hand, if you are in your thirties and have a 50° curve, but your curve has not progressed since adolescence, and you experience no back pain, surgery would probably not be appropriate—at least not yet.

Your curve is progressing. Regardless of the current degree measurement, most surgeons would agree that a patient who has a curve with a demonstrated history of progression is a viable surgical candidate. This is especially true if the patient is very young (because curvatures can progress rapidly until maturity) or if the curve has already progressed beyond 50° (because the probability is high that the curve will continue to progress).

Young patients who have not yet finished growing and whose curves are less than about 40° will typically be braced. If bracing treatment is not a viable option or is not successful, your orthopedist will consider surgery.

You have severe or chronic back pain attributed to scoliosis. Regardless of the measurement of the curve, if scoliosis can be pinpointed as the cause of severe or chronic pain, surgery should be considered. However, conventional pain management techniques should always be tried first. This includes medications, exercise, physical therapy, back supports, changes in lifestyle, new furniture, and other more conservative approaches to pain management. You should understand that scoliosis surgery provides no guarantee that your pain will be alleviated. Approximately 80% of adults report a "significant" reduction in pain after surgery. That means that one in five patients still has some level of pain postoperatively. It is also possible that the location or nature of the pain will change; for example, your mid-back may feel better, but your shoulder may hurt more.

Even if any of the above applies to you, there are some important *contraindications* for scoliosis surgery—reasons you would not be a viable candidate, or at least not at this time. These include:

You are too old. The health risks of performing any surgery on an older adult may not be justified. Surgeons differ on their opinions of how old is too old; it varies by patient, but 60-70 years old is a common threshold. As you age, bones become increasingly brittle due to osteoporosis and other conditions, discs degenerate, and the spine's natural flexibility diminishes. These factors mean that the level of correction achievable is lower than in a younger patient, and the risk of complications is higher. Coupled with the surgical risks of anesthesia and the difficult recovery process, surgery for older individuals is seldom a good prospect.

You are in frail health. Scoliosis surgery stresses your body. You need to be in relatively good health to be able to minimize the risks associated with the surgery and to enjoy a relatively quick and safe recovery. Remember that scoliosis surgery is never emergency surgery that must be performed urgently. If you have an illness that can be treated, first pursue appropriate treatment for it before considering scoliosis surgery.

You are an addicted smoker and are unwilling to quit. Nicotine reduces the probability that a good fusion will occur because it interferes with the body's ability to form new bone. Use of a nicotine patch or gum is no safer.

In a study of patients who underwent cervical fusion, smokers had an increased rate of fusion failure (up to 47%) compared to non-smokers.[1] Another study evaluated tobacco use in patients who underwent lumbar fusion. The patients who smoked had failed fusions in up to 40% of cases, compared to only 8% among non-smokers.[2] Yet another study showed that cigarette smoking compromises the immune system, which can increase the patient's susceptibility to postoperative infection.[3] For these reasons, many surgeons will not perform a spinal fusion on someone who smokes.

Incidentally, there is some research to support that smoking may exacerbate back pain, particularly in individuals with scoliosis. If reducing chronic back pain is one of your primary motivations to have scoliosis surgery, you may want to cease smoking for a while to see if the pain subsides.

Your primary objective is to improve your cosmetic appearance. You might be interested in surgery to improve physical deformities caused by scoliosis, such as a rib hump, uneven shoulders, or poor posture. Indeed, these kinds of aesthetic issues can be improved or corrected by surgery. However, unless your deformity is truly severe, it is difficult to justify taking on the risks and agonizing recovery of surgery merely to improve your appearance, especially if you are not experiencing any pain or your curvature is not progressing. Few surgeons would perform surgery in such a case.

You have no support system for recovery. Chapter 4 will explore the importance of having a reliable support system during the recovery period. If no family members or friends are available to help you, and you cannot afford a private nurse to assist you, you might want to delay surgery until your situation changes. Alternatively, some patients feel that they can handle the recovery process on their own, and some do, in fact, tackle it successfully.

The Goals of Surgery

There are three primary objectives to spinal fusion:

1. *To prevent further curve progression.* The curvature of a spine that has been surgically fused will rarely progress more than 5° or so for the remainder of the patient's life.

2. *To reduce—though not completely eliminate—the curvature and rotation.* A common misconception is that scoliosis surgery corrects curvatures to 0° with no rotation, which is another way of saying "perfectly straight." This is possible in only an extremely small percentage of cases. More typically, using modern surgical techniques and instrumentation, the reduction in curvature will be in the range of 60-90% and the rotation will be almost, though rarely completely, eliminated. See *Estimating Correction.*

    Note that correction of a scoliotic curve is not always a goal of the surgery. In some extreme situations, efforts to correct the curvature would not produce a good surgical outcome and may present unacceptable risks to the patient. In these cases, the goal may be limited merely to stabilizing the spine to prevent further curve progression (the first point above).

3. *To relieve pain caused by scoliosis.* As mentioned previously, not all patients experience pain related to their curvatures. For those who do, surgery *may* reduce or eliminate the pain. Studies of the effectiveness of spinal fusion as a means of eliminating pain show effectiveness rates of 65-80%. Then again, to some extent, the surgery is analogous to preventive maintenance for those who are not currently experiencing pain, as pain associated with scoliosis tends to increase with the patient's age.

Without exception, you should have a very honest discussion with your surgeon about your expectations of the surgery and his or her assessment of the likelihood of meeting those expectations. You need to be clear on expected outcomes in order to make an informed choice about proceeding with surgery.

Overview of the Surgical Procedure

Scoliosis surgery is really two procedures in one, and you should understand the difference. One aspect of the surgery involves *fusing* certain vertebrae, while the other part involves attaching stabilizing hardware, called *instrumentation*, to those vertebrae. This is why the clinical name for scoliosis surgery is *spinal fusion with instrumentation.*

The word *fusion* means "to bring together." The goal of fusing vertebrae is to transform the misaligned vertebrae into a single, solid block of bone that will not increase in curvature over time. Fusing a spine is not what you might expect; it is not fusion in the sense of welding, such as by melting bone with heat. Instead, the surgeon strips away the outer bone of certain vertebrae, exposing the porous living bone underneath. This living bone has a rich blood supply and thus will bleed. Your body reacts to this as if it were dealing with a fracture. To heal itself, your body will flood the stripped-away area of vertebrae with blood that contains new bone-forming cells.

To help the vertebrae fuse into a stronger, more solid piece of bone, the surgeon will mix-in small strips or crushed pieces of bone from elsewhere in your body or from another source. This is called *bone grafting.* Over time, new bone is formed. The new bone will not resemble normal, flexible vertebrae;

rather, it will be a single, solid block of bone that spans the length of the exposed vertebrae.

Spinal fusion alone will not hold a scoliotic curve. The fusion process
takes at least six months to one year until the new bone is fully formed and
rigid. During that time, the spine will continue to move, and therefore there is
no assurance that your spine will heal in a straightened position. This is no
different than any other bone fracture in the body. If you break your arm, for
example, the bone will heal on its own but you must wear a cast to keep the
bone immobilized so that it heals in the correct position. In the same way,
your spine needs to be stabilized during the healing process. To do this, your
surgeon will attach hardware (*instrumentation*) to the vertebrae that were fused.
This is called *internal fixation* (internal because the hardware is inside your
body, fixation because the hardware fixates, or holds, your bones).

Surgical Approaches

Scoliosis surgery obviously requires that the surgeon be able to access your
spine. How he or she does this is called an *approach*. An incision can either be
made on your back side (a *posterior approach*), from your front and side (*anterior*), or a combination of the two. In addition, there is a newer procedure
called the *endoscopic* or *thoracoscopic approach*, which is described later in this
chapter.

The posterior approach is the most common and is generally used for
patients with flexible thoracic or thoracolumbar curves. Posterior-approach
surgeries typically have fewer complications than anterior-approach surgeries
because no organs need to be moved out of the way during the procedure.
Because of this, patients will generally have a posterior-approach surgery
unless there is a specific benefit or medical reason to perform it anteriorly.
The only downside of the posterior approach is cosmetic: it leaves a long
scar.

The anterior approach is generally used on younger patients with flexible
thoracolumbar or lumbar curves, older patients with very stiff curves, or patients with significant sagittal curve deformities (flatback or hunchback). It
may also be performed on patients with a thoracic curve, but there is rarely a
benefit in doing this over a posterior approach.

Whether the anterior approach is superior to the posterior approach is debatable. Proponents of the anterior approach argue that it results in better levels of correction for thoracolumbar and lumbar curves, requires that fewer lumbar vertebrae be fused, and that it offers faster recovery times and less pain for patients. However, a 1999 study did not provide compelling support for these assertions, and simultaneously revealed some disturbing outcomes.[4] The study indeed found that an average of 2.5 fewer lumbar levels could be saved (not fused) in an anterior surgery versus an equivalent posterior surgery. However, the complication rate was alarmingly higher for the patients who underwent anterior surgeries: 23% of patients who had anterior surgeries lost more than 10° of correction after their surgery, versus only 11% of those who had posterior surgeries. *Pseudarthrosis* (failure of the vertebrae to fuse successfully) was also five times more common in the anterior group (5% of patients, versus 1% for posterior surgeries). The hardware broke in 31% of the anterior patients but in only 1% of the posterior patients. Some of these high complication rates may be explained by the particular type of hardware consistently used in the anterior surgeries. With newer types of hardware and better surgeon training, these problems have allegedly become rare.

Since the late 1990s, posterior-approach surgical techniques and instrumentation have also improved, effectively closing the gap between the commonly cited benefits of anterior approaches over posterior approaches. Using new forms of instrumentation, particularly pedicle screws to attach rods to the spine instead of the more conventional hooks, the amount of correction achievable and the number of vertebrae that need to be fused are now approximately equal between the two types of surgeries. Given the higher complication rate of anterior surgeries, it is difficult to justify its superiority over posterior approaches.

Even so, there are still some specific situations in which the anterior approach is clearly preferred, such as surgeries limited to the lumbar area, where saving even one level can make a substantial difference in a patient's flexibility. Your surgeon will select the surgical approach that he or she feels is most suitable in your case. Surgeons will also base this decision, in part, on the approach they are most comfortable performing and with which they have observed the best results. A good surgeon can achieve an excellent result using either technique.

Posterior-Approach Surgery

As with any scoliosis surgery, you will first be put under general anesthesia. You will not remember any of the following.

You will be placed on the operating table facing down, in what is called the prone position. This position (Figure 7) is the most commonly used for posterior-approach surgeries. Note the supporting pads underneath the torso and thighs. After surgery, some patients have mild soreness in these areas from prolonged pressure.

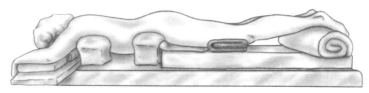

Figure 7: The prone position

An incision will be made down the middle of your back (called a *midline incision*), over the spine. The length of the incision depends on how many vertebrae the surgeon intends to fuse. The incision is usually between six and fourteen inches long. The surgeon will then open the incision and strip away all tissue surrounding the area to be fused so that he or she can access your spine (Figure 8).

In many cases, the surgeon will then cut away the facet joints (see Figure 2 in Chapter 1) from the portion of spine that will be fused. Removing the facet joints makes the spine more flexible, which enables the surgeon to more freely adjust the spine into the desired position prior to fusion.

With the spine now fully exposed, the surgeon will add the instrumentation. There are three basic types of instrumentation the surgeon can use to affix the rods to your spine: hooks, pedicle screws, and wires. A hook "grabs on" to your spine in the open space of your spinal canal, or can be affixed to the transverse processes (the bony projections on the sides of your vertebrae) or to the facet joints. A pedicle screw literally screws into the pedicle of your vertebrae.

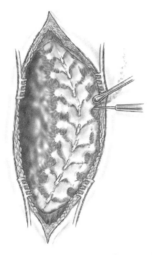

Figure 8: Opening the incision and exposing the spine

The decision to use hooks or pedicle screws—or both, in different places on your spine—depends on a variety of factors. Screws are generally stronger and more securely mounted than hooks, and thus will tolerate a greater degree of corrective force; that is, your surgeon may be able to straighten your spine more by using screws rather than hooks. Hooks, however, are easier and faster to place, and are generally considered safer to use than screws, which must be drilled into your spine very close to your spinal cord.

Some surgeons prefer to place screws only in the lumbar region, because the lumbar vertebrae are larger and thus placing screws in them is relatively straightforward. The vertebrae higher in your back are smaller, so some surgeons prefer to use hooks in these areas. Still other surgeons use pedicle screws throughout a spine. Other factors can influence this decision. For example, using pedicle screws may not be possible if your vertebrae are weak or brittle. The most important thing for you to know is that a good surgeon can achieve an excellent surgical outcome with either hooks or screws.

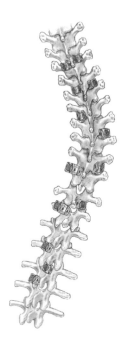

Figure 9: Hooks positioned along the spine prior to attaching rods

Before rods can be attached to the pedicle screws or hooks, they must be gently contoured to follow the natural sagittal (front-to-back) curves of your spine. This is done using a tool called a bender (Figure 10). Your surgeon might instead use a rod that is pre-contoured.

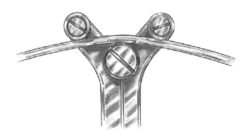

Figure 10: Bending (contouring) a rod

The contoured rods are then attached to the screws or hooks using various connectors. Then, to straighten your spine, a surgeon can use a variety of tools to adjust the forces the rods exert on your spine in three dimensions (Figure 11). Most scoliotic spines are rotated about their axis. The surgeon therefore will "crank" the rods to de-rotate your spine so that it is straight from side-to-side (laterally). The surgeon also can adjust the forces on the rods to preserve the normal sagittal curves.

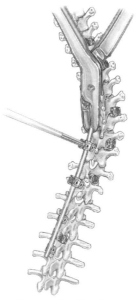

Figure 11: Attaching and adjusting a contoured rod

In addition to the two rods (one on each side of your spine), additional instrumentation components, called *transverse connectors* or *cross-links*, are bridged between the two parallel rods. These give the rods added structural rigidity. The connectors attach only to the rods, not to your spine. Two connectors are used: one is placed high between the rods and one is placed low. The result is that the rods and connectors roughly form a tall rectangle.

Once the hooks or screws are secured to the spine, the surgeon will initiate the fusion process by scraping (*decorticating*) the surface of the vertebrae in the area to be fused. This will cause the vertebrae to bleed, though the total amount of blood loss is typically modest. The surgeon will mix-in small chips of bone grafting material to the bleeding area as fusion material. This area is called the *fusion bed*. In some cases a surgeon will create the fusion bed prior to adding pedicle screws or affixing hooks.

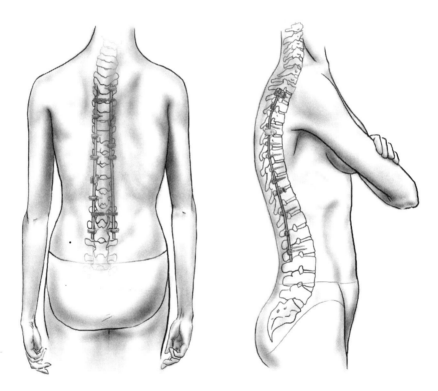

**Figure 12: Typical posterior-approach
segmental instrumentation in place**

After all the hardware is adjusted and your spine is straightened as much and as safely as the surgeon deems possible, your incision will be closed and you will be taken to the recovery room. The final result will resemble that shown in Figure 12.

Anterior-Approach Surgeries

In an anterior-approach surgery, you will be placed on the operating table on your side (Figure 13). An incision will be made beginning on your side and continuing down and toward the front of your body. Because your arm will cover part of the incision, the resulting scar will be less noticeable than in a posterior-approach surgery.

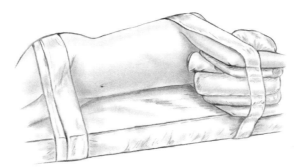

Figure 13: Typical positioning for an anterior-approach surgery

For anterior surgeries higher in the back, the surgeon may need to deflate one of your lungs, temporarily detach the diaphragm, and remove a rib to gain access to the spine. The rib will often be used for bone grafting material and will grow back within a few months. For surgeries limited to the lower back, these steps may be skipped.

Deflation of a lung can be risky. While under anesthesia, your breathing must be entirely supported by one lung. In the controlled environment of an operating room, this is rarely a problem for healthy individuals, but those who have a history of smoking, asthma, or another lung condition may not be able to tolerate this aspect of the procedure. For these patients, a posterior-approach surgery may be the best option.

In anterior surgeries, most surgeons will remove the discs between vertebrae in the area to be fused, a procedure called a *discectomy*. By removing the discs, the surgeon can pack in more bone grafting material between the vertebrae, and can more freely adjust the spine prior to fusion.

The final steps of installing instrumentation and creating the fusion bed are similar to that in the posterior approach, except it is of course being done from your side, not your back.

Combined Anterior/Posterior Approaches

A combination of anterior and posterior approaches (denoted *A/P* or called *circumferential fusion*) is another surgical option. In this hybrid technique, the lumbar curve is usually accessed anteriorly, while the thoracic curve is reached posteriorly. Instrumentation is usually only added to the posterior side. The surgeon will typically complete the procedure on one side and then move on to the other, but in some cases the surgeon will go back and forth between the two sides in what is called a *540 degree sequence*. This is also called a *front-back-front* (anterior-posterior-anterior) or *back-front-back* (posterior-anterior-posterior) approach. The A/P approach may be indicated if any of the following conditions apply:

- You have a severe structural curve of 70° or more (some surgeons would say 60°, some would say 75°)
- Your curve is rigid, as determined by analyzing bending films (see *Estimating Correction*)
- You are at least 60 years old. Older patients have a higher risk of pseudarthrosis, which is reduced if the spine is fused anteriorly and posteriorly.
- The patient is under 10 years old. In young, rapidly-growing children, the curvature of the anterior portion of the spine would continue to progress even if the posterior portion were fused. This is called the *crankshaft effect*.
- Your sagittal curves are unbalanced. If your lower back is too flat (too little lordosis) or your upper back too hunchback (severe kyphosis), an A/P approach can help restore these normal curves.
- You need a long fusion down to the sacrum
- Your scoliosis is caused by a neuromuscular disorder
- The surgery is a revision case (see *Longer-Term Surgical Risks and Complications*)

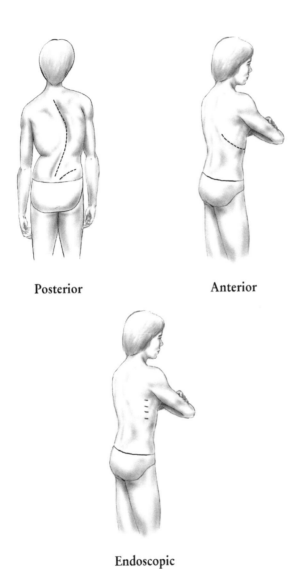

Posterior   Anterior

Endoscopic

Figure 14: Typical incision sites for each approach. The smaller scar on the posterior-approach illustration would only be made if bone grafting material were being harvested from the pelvis.

Anterior/posterior surgery is a long procedure—often lasting up to twelve hours. Some surgeons will divide the procedure over two days, which may be scheduled days or weeks apart. It is usually preferable if your surgeon can perform both approaches in the same surgical session. The primary benefit of a single operation is a faster recovery due to less anesthesia and thus a shorter hospital stay (as little as five days versus up to two weeks). Psychological trauma is also reduced by having one rather than two surgeries. The potential disadvantages include excessive blood loss, severe pressure sores, and higher neurological risks. You should discuss these issues with your surgeon if you have been told that you may be required to undergo A/P surgery.

The Thoracoscopic/Endoscopic Approach

In this minimally-invasive technique, interchangeably called *thoracoscopic* or *endoscopic approaches*, the spine is accessed through several small incisions in the side of the chest instead of one large incision in the back or front. The surgeon inserts a device called an *endoscope*—an instrument with a tiny fiberoptic video camera and light at one end—into the incisions to observe your spine. Instruments are then inserted through the small incisions, called *portals* (Figure 15), to perform the fusion, insert instrumentation, and remove discs, if necessary. The thoracoscopic approach is primarily employed on individuals with the following characteristics:

- A single thoracic curve measuring between 40° and 80° (some surgeons would select 60° as an upper limit), or a thoracolumbar curve where the lumbar curve is relatively small and thus only a selective thoracic fusion is appropriate
- A highly flexible spine. This usually means younger patients.
- A kyphotic curve of less than 40° (some surgeons would say less than 20°). Anterior instrumentation tends to increase kyphosis, so the lower this measurement, the better.

This technique is generally not used on patients whose scoliosis is associated with neuromuscular disease, those who have a high degree of kyphosis, or those who cannot tolerate one-lung anesthesia. One lung must be completely collapsed during the procedure to allow space for the endoscope and other instruments.

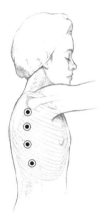

Figure 15: Portal placement for endoscopic-approach surgeries

There are several potential benefits of the thoracoscopic approach over the standard posterior and anterior approaches, including:

- Fewer fused vertebrae. This may result in less correction but more flexibility.
- Shorter hospital stays—as little as three days
- Less blood loss during surgery
- Faster recovery, with less pain
- Less noticeable scars

A 1996-1998 study of fifty patients with thoracic curves yielded promising results.[5] These patients had thoracoscopic fusions with instrumentation. Key results included:

- The first forty patients averaged corrections of 50.2%, while the final ten averaged 68.6%, presumably due to improved skills developed by the surgeons with increasing experience

- Postoperative pain was less, and the patients were off pain medications within one to three weeks, as opposed to six to twelve weeks for those who had traditional surgeries
- Hospital stays averaged three days. Five to seven days is more typical for traditional approaches.

Surgical complications are more common with thoracoscopic techniques. In particular, the rate of pseudarthrosis is high relative to those who have traditional "open" posterior or anterior surgeries. One spine surgeon estimates that the pseudarthrosis rate for thoracoscopic surgeries may exceed 30% for unskilled surgeons and 10-15% for more skilled surgeons. Other surgical complications are not uncommon. In the study of fifty patients, fourteen developed complications, though none were life threatening and all were correctable. In another study of thirty patients, two patients developed temporary leg paralysis, three patients accumulated fluid in their lungs, and the rods in three patients broke after surgery.[6] Fortunately, the complication rate for thoracoscopic surgeries is dropping over time as surgeons become more skilled in these techniques.

In addition to a higher-than-normal complication rate, another downside of this approach is that it requires patients to be exposed to numerous x-rays during surgery. Because surgeons perform their work via video camera rather than by direct observation, frequent *intraoperative* (actions taken during surgery) x-rays are necessary to verify that the desired results are being obtained. It is not clear whether this level of exposure to x-ray radiation is harmful, but it is certainly a risk worth noting.

You might want to ask your surgeon whether the endoscopic approach would be appropriate in your case. Keep in mind, however, that this technique is still considered somewhat experimental, no long-term data on its outcome is available, and few surgeons have experience performing this technique.

Bone Grafting Options

As mentioned previously, during surgery your surgeon will mix in additional bone matter to your exposed vertebrae to facilitate faster and more rigid healing. The surgeon can source this bone from three different types of material.

Autograft, also called *autogenous*. The most common source of bone grafting material is bone taken from the patient's own body during surgery. This is usually harvested from the top of the pelvic bone, called the *iliac crest*, or from a rib. Patients who are also having thoracoplasty performed (explained in the next section) or who are having anterior-approach surgeries higher in the back will most likely have bone removed from the ribs instead of the pelvis, since both require the removal of some amount of rib as part of the procedure. In addition, it is sometimes possible to remove chips of bone from other parts of the spine as it being worked on (called *local bone grafting*). Almost all posterior-approach surgeries will utilize autografts.

Autografts have excellent fusion rates, and there is no risk that the body will reject the graft since it came from the patient's own body. There are some disadvantages, however. One is that the patient may experience postoperative pain or numbness in the area where the bone was removed. In addition, the step of removing bone increases both the amount of blood lost during surgery and the amount of time under anesthesia.

Harvesting bone from the pelvis instead of a rib presents two unique problems. First, a separate incision may need to be made to access the hip, thus resulting in a second scar. A second and more important risk is the possibility of chronic, long-term (and sometimes permanent) pain in the area of the hip graft. Research varies in how common this is, but as many as 31% of patients studied report having some pain in the area of their hip graft months or even years after surgery, though few rate this pain as severe.[7] Because of this, some surgeons now exclusively rely on the ribs as a source of autograft material. However, some adult patients report significant pain in the area of their rib grafts for up to two years after surgery.

Allograft, also called *bone-bank bone* or *donor bone*. This is bone taken from a deceased person who has consented to donate his or her organs for transplant purposes after death. Allograft bone is extensively tested and processed to ensure that it is safe to use in patients. Almost all anterior-approach surgeries will require some allograft bone because more grafting material is needed for this type of surgery than can be obtained safely from the patient by autograft. Allografts may also be required if the patient has had prior bone grafts that depleted the necessary reserves of autograft bone material.

The advantages of allografts complement the disadvantages of autografts: less pain, less blood loss and time under anesthesia, and no separate incision. However, there are potentially serious drawbacks. Studies have shown that using allograft bone as the only graft material results in poor fusion rates in the thoracic and lumbar regions. There is also a greater probability of rejection. For larger fusion areas a mixture of allograft bone and autograft bone can be an effective solution.

A variant of traditional allograft bone is called demineralized bone matrix (DBM). Some of the proteins that stimulate bone formation are extracted (demineralized) from bone taken from a cadaver. The proteins are then transformed into various forms—usually a gel—that can be added to a graft site to enhance fusion. Currently, DBM is only used to supplement, not completely replace, autograft or regular allograft bone.

Bone morphogenetic protein (BMP, or rhBMP-2) is found naturally in the human body and stimulates bone formation by transforming "regular" cells into bone-forming cells. BMP can be used to supplement autografts or allografts, or in some cases can be used exclusively.

BMP increases the likelihood of a successful fusion, and it accelerates the rate at which the fusion process takes place. In one 1997 study, 10 out of 11 patients who underwent spinal fusions using BMP achieved successful fusions within only three months of surgery. In contrast, most fusions using allograft or autograft bone take at least a full year to heal completely.

If BMP is used in lieu of autograft bone, an additional benefit to patients may be less postoperative pain (because no bone has been removed) and a faster recovery time (because the patient would be under anesthesia for less time without the added surgical step of bone grafting).

Though used experimentally for several years, the U.S. Food and Drug Administration only approved BMP in 2002 for limited use in spine surgery. This approval covered the use of BMP in single-level anterior fusions low in the back, and only when used in conjunction with special titanium "cages" that surround the spine and hold something like a sponge soaked in BMP. Nonetheless, some surgeons are experimenting with the use of BMP in other circumstances.

BMP is extremely expensive, and most insurance companies will not cover its use. Furthermore, no long-term studies on its effectiveness are available. For these reasons, few surgeons use BMP today, and the number of patients on which it has been used is still relatively small. Still, BMP may someday eliminate the need for bone grafting.

Thoracoplasty (Rib Hump Removal)

A complementary surgical procedure your surgeon may recommend is called *thoracoplasty*. This is a procedure to flatten the rib hump that affects most scoliosis patients with a thoracic curve (Figure 16). It may also be done to obtain bone grafts from the ribs instead of the pelvis, regardless of whether a rib hump is present.

Thoracoplasty is the removal (or *resection*) of typically four to six segments of adjacent ribs that protrude. Each segment is one to two inches long. The surgeon decides which ribs to resect based on either their prominence or by identifying which ribs are unlikely to be realigned by correction of the curvature alone. Thoracoplasty does not involve the removal of entire ribs, just sections of them. Amazingly, ribs grow back and, when they do, they will grow back straight. The newly-grown ribs are usually just as strong as the original ribs.

There are two significant benefits of thoracoplasty. The first is a better cosmetic appearance. Your rib hump will be flattened, providing you with a smoother back and a more natural appearance. Clothing will drape better around your shoulder blades. Leaning back on chairs will feel more comfortable, as your back will not protrude as much.

The second benefit is also cosmetic: you may have one less scar. Recall that spinal fusion requires bone for grafting material. If your surgeon performs a posterior-approach procedure and chooses to use autograft material, he or she has two places from which to obtain it: your pelvis or your ribs. Taking bone from the pelvis may require making a second incision low in the back, thus resulting in a second scar. However, bone can always be taken from the section of ribs resected in thoracoplasty through the same midline incision (down the middle of your back) that the surgeon will make to access your spine, though some surgeons prefer to make a second incision over the peak of the rib hump. In a sense, thoracoplasty kills two birds with one stone—you get a more natural-looking back while potentially avoiding a second scar.

Related to the second benefit is that bone grafts taken from the ribs typically cause less long-term pain for the patient than grafts taken from the pelvis. Furthermore, although most patients with a rib hump do not experience pain from the hump itself, if you do have pain in the hump area, thoracoplasty can help eliminate this.

Thoracoplasty has risks and complications. The most significant drawback is increased pain in the rib area during recovery. Indeed, you will experience postoperative pain regardless of whether thoracoplasty is performed, but this procedure will heighten the pain in the specific areas where your ribs were resected. If you have ever had a broken rib, you know roughly what this feels like. Ribs can take two to three months to heal.

Another complication is temporarily reduced pulmonary function following surgery. A 10-15% reduction in pulmonary function is typical. You will probably find it harder to take deep breaths and may become "winded" more easily than usual. This impairment can last anywhere from a few months to two years. Patients with asthma or other respiratory problems should discuss this issue with their surgeon, though it is usually not problematic.

Because thoracoplasty may lengthen the duration of the surgery, you may also lose more blood or develop complications from the prolonged anesthesia. A more significant, though far less common risk is that the surgeon will inadvertently puncture your *pleura*, a protective coating over the lungs. This could cause blood or air to drain into your chest cavity, conditions called a *hemothorax* or *pneumothorax*, respectively. To remove excess blood, a chest tube would need to be inserted for two to three days, which is uncomfortable but usually not painful. A pneumothorax may cause one of your lungs to deflate, but this can be remedied in a controlled hospital setting relatively easily. Some pneumothorax conditions will repair themselves without endangering the patient.

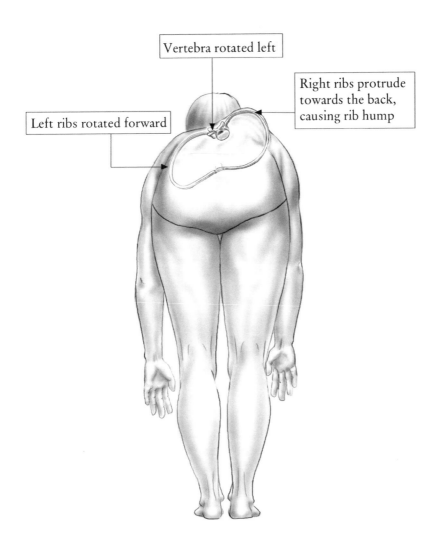

Vertebra rotated left

Right ribs protrude towards the back, causing rib hump

Left ribs rotated forward

Figure 16: Typical structure of a rib hump

Surgeons differ in their opinions on the effect of wearing a brace after surgery (see *Postoperative Bracing* in Chapter 6). Some feel it may reduce the risk of a hemothorax by preventing the ribs from rubbing against the chest cavity. Others argue that wearing a brace may actually cause a hemothorax to develop more easily by making deep breathing more difficult.

If you are not sure you want thoracoplasty, you could initially undergo spinal fusion and note the effect this has on your rib hump. You can always have thoracoplasty later, after a fusion. This will, of course, result in additional pain, cost, time, and trouble, and every time you have surgery there are risks. Therefore, if you think you will ever have thoracoplasty, it is better to have it done at the same time as your fusion. Note that undergoing thoracoplasty without having a spinal fusion will yield no benefit. The resected ribs will grow back crooked if the underlying spinal curvature and rotation is not first reduced.

Estimating Correction

You will of course want to know how much of your curvature can be corrected with scoliosis surgery. The truth is, no surgeon can accurately predict this. But you can get a reasonably good ballpark estimation using a tool called *bending x-rays* (or *bending films*). The best predictor of how much your curve can be corrected is an analysis of the natural flexibility in your spine. Bending films provide insight into this level of flexibility.

A bending film is an x-ray picture of your back, taken from above you while you are lying down, face-up (called the *supine position*) and bending as far as possible to one side. X-rays will typically be taken of you bending both to your right and to your left. A Cobb angle of your spinal curvature in these positions is then calculated. This measurement is a rough predictor of to what degree your curve can be corrected. The logic behind this is straightforward. Suppose you have a 60° right thoracic curve, measured standing up. If that same curve measures 30° when you bend hard to your right, this would indicate that your vertebrae in the thoracic region are flexible enough to correct 30° with some force. Spinal fusion and instrumentation will simulate this same force.

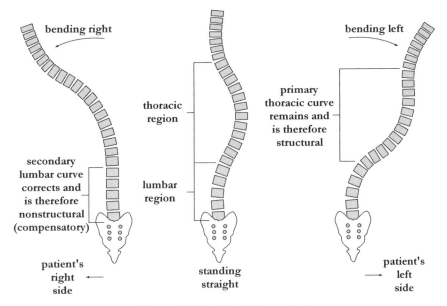

Figure 17: Bending film analysis

A high degree of flexibility is key to large corrections. With age, the flexibility of the vertebrae decreases. This is why young patients, with plenty of flexibility in their spines, can achieve very high levels of correction from scoliosis surgery. It is also why very old patients may not get much correction at all, which is important for these patients to take into account when deciding to have surgery. In general, the younger you are, the more flexible your spine is, and the more correction you can achieve.

Other factors must be considered in predicting the amount of correction attainable in your particular case. Your surgeon will rely on his or her training, gut feelings, and experience to give you a rough estimate. Some generalities can be made, but again, every scoliosis case is unique and your results may vary. In general:

- *The younger the patient, the better the correction.* Statistically, the amount of correction achievable in teenagers and young adults averages 50-60%, whereas in adults the average is closer to 40%. You may achieve far better or worse than these figures depending on a variety of factors.

- *Surgeries that exclusively use pedicle screws typically result in better correction.* The exclusive use of pedicle screw instrumentation generally results in better correction levels—on average, about 80%—than any combination of hooks and wires, or combinations that incorporate some pedicle screws. Note, though, that pedicle screws are not appropriate in all surgical cases. See *Surgical Instrumentation.*

- *Anterior-approach surgery typically results in better correction than posterior-approach surgery for lumbar curves.* On average, anterior surgery typically results in 70-80% correction in younger people and 50% correction in adults.

- *Single structural curves are easier to correct than multiple structural curves*

Achieving 100% correction is seldom possible, for three reasons. First, the vertebrae that comprise the structural curve of a severe scoliotic spine are often physically deformed. No amount of fusion or instrumentation can perfectly re-align them. Second, if a surgeon exerts too much force on your spine in an effort to straighten it, your vertebrae could actually fracture, or you could end up with neurological damage to your spinal column. The third reason is the risk of *decompensation.* As mentioned earlier, many cases of scoliosis have a structural curve and one or two compensatory curves. If a structural curve is corrected too much, the compensatory curves may not be able to counter-balance the degree of curvature remaining. The result is that the patient may be a little off-center, leaning slightly to one side.

Bending films are also useful in differentiating structural curves from compensatory, or nonstructural, curves (see Figure 17). Simply put, if bending hard in one direction causes a section of your spine that appears crooked when standing upright to suddenly become straight, that curve is compensatory. Compensatory curves usually straighten significantly on their own when structural curves are corrected, but seldom correct 100%. In contrast, curves that do not correct much (or not at all) on bending films are rigid and therefore structural. Most surgeons consider any curve that does not "bend out" to less than 25° to be structural. This means that, for example, a curve that measures 60° on a standing P/A x-ray and 30° on a bending film would still be considered structural, even though the curve exhibits enough flexibility to correct 50%.

Impact on Flexibility

You are surely interested to know whether fusing your spine will limit your flexibility. Will you still be able to bend over? Bend to your side? Arch your back? Without question, scoliosis surgery will limit your ability to do all these things *somewhat*, but the extent to which your flexibility is limited will vary based on what specific vertebrae are fused. Not every one of the twenty-four vertebra in your spine are involved equally in your ability to bend your back.

Your five lumbar vertebrae (L1-L5) are the most important for maintaining flexibility. Every surgeon will try to avoid fusing these vertebrae if possible, though fusing just L1 will not have a significant impact on one's flexibility. Some lumbar deformities are so severe, however, that a surgeon must fuse "down to the sacrum"—fusing all five lumbar levels and anchoring the instrumentation to the sacrum. Adolescents are rarely fused to the sacrum, whereas adults are sometimes fused to the sacrum when there is severe disc degeneration between the lower end of the curve and the sacrum. Fusing to the sacrum will, unfortunately, result in a substantial loss of bending flexibility.

The seven cervical vertebrae are the second most important area in terms of flexibility. Spinal fusions for correcting scoliosis rarely fuse vertebrae high in the neck, but even the lower cervical vertebrae are substantially involved in your ability to bend and rotate your neck.

The twelve thoracic vertebrae are the least important to bending flexibility. Because these vertebrae support the rib cage, they do not bend much even in a normal spine. A fusion limited to the thoracic region will therefore not result in significant bending limitations.

People who have had spinal fusions learn to compensate for reductions in flexibility. They bend more with the other, non-fused sections of their spine, and they bend more from their hips and use their legs to get closer to the ground. Your overall flexibility may be diminished, but your functional ability to continue doing the things you want to do is not usually as reduced as you might expect.

Surgical Instrumentation

Your surgeon may choose from a large array of hardware (instrumentation) to fixate your spine—rods, screws, hooks, cross-links, wires, and other hardware. These come in all kinds of sizes, shapes, materials, and strengths. As a patient, you do not need to delve deeply into learning about all the options from which your surgeon can choose—*if you trust your surgeon*. This section addresses what you really need to know.

Harrington Rods versus Segmental Systems

Harrington rods are rarely used today—in fact, almost never in more developed countries. As you research scoliosis, you may uncover horror stories about Harrington rods from people who had scoliosis surgery in the 1980s or earlier. At that time, the Harrington rod was the only surgical option. Harrington rods, named after the orthopedic surgeon who invented them, are predecessors to the newer type of rods used in almost every surgery today. In the old surgical technique, a single Harrington rod was attached to the top and bottom end-points of the concave side of a scoliotic curve. The rod forced the curve to straighten by pulling those end-points farther apart from each other.

Suffice to say, surgery with Harrington rods was nowhere near as effective as modern surgical techniques. Patients typically had to wear a cast for months after surgery, correction levels were not particularly high, good lumbar correction was not achievable, and it was not at all uncommon for these rods to break off the vertebrae to which they were attached years after surgery. Many patients needed additional surgery later due to broken rods or flatback syndrome.

In the 1960s and 1970s, so-called "second generation systems" were introduced as improvements or alternatives to a Harrington rod. One of these techniques, called Luque after its inventor, placed two rods on either side of the spine that were attached to the spine using wires. Correction levels were not particularly high, and the risk of damage to the spinal canal through which the wires passed was significant. Though rare, similar "sublaminar wiring" techniques are still used today for patients whose bones are too fragile for hooks and screws, or for those whose scoliosis is caused by problems with their nerves and muscles.

Introduced in the 1980s and continuing through to the present day, *segmental systems* are the instrumentation of choice. These are also called *third generation systems*. You may come across names like C-D (Cotrel-Dubousset; the two doctors who invented third generation systems), TSRH® (Texas Scottish Rite Hospital), ISOLA®, or Moss Miami™. Each system differs mainly in how the hooks or pedicle screws affix to the rods using different kinds of connectors. It is unnecessary to be concerned with the specifics of those to be used in your surgery.

Unlike Harrington rods, segmental rods can be attached at multiple points to multiple vertebrae ("segments") using a variety of hardware (hooks, screws, and wires, in any combination). This flexibility has resulted in a wealth of benefits: better correction, better postoperative balance and posture, and higher rates of successful fusions. In addition, patients now rarely need to wear a brace postoperatively (though some surgeons still recommend it).

In the unlikely event that your surgeon wants to use Harrington rods, be sure to question why, and by all means seek a second opinion. A small number of surgeons still use Harrington rods, not because they are a superior system (they clearly are not), but rather because that is what they were trained to use long ago and are thus the most comfortable using. Because Harrington rods are an obsolete technology and therefore inexpensive relative to more modern instruments, they are still occasionally used in less developed nations.

Stainless Steel versus Titanium Rods

As you research scoliosis, you may encounter debate over the pros and cons of stainless steel versus titanium rods. Neither one stands out as superior to the other. The key benefit of titanium is that it will not distort MRI (magnetic resonance imaging) scans of your spine taken after surgery, if they ever need to be taken. Titanium is also lighter. But stainless steel is stronger than titanium, and far less expensive. Some insurance companies will not cover the use of titanium instrumentation.

Both titanium and stainless steel have unique risks. Titanium rods may exhibit something called "metal memory." A 2005 study found that if titanium rods are contoured at room temperature (for example, in an operating room) and then maintained at a constant body temperature, over time the rods may gradually revert to their original shape. This can result in loss of sagittal balance or pedicle screw pullout.[8]

There is also a risk of having an allergic reaction to the nickel contained in stainless steel rods. This will generally only occur if a rod is damaged and is "shedding" particles into your body. As much as 15% of the U.S. population is allergic to nickel. Prolonged exposure to nickel can cause pain and internal bleeding, necessitating that the rods be removed. You may have experienced this if you have ever had body piercings. If you have any reason to believe you are allergic to nickel, you should be tested for this before having surgery, or ask your surgeon to use titanium rods.

Removal of Hardware

In most cases, hardware *can* be removed after at least one year has lapsed since surgery (some surgeons recommend waiting as many as five years). Recall that the hardware is only there to stabilize your spine until the fusion process is complete. Most patients do not experience any problems with, let alone notice, their hardware after a few months. Removing the hardware is therefore only appropriate in the following cases:

- There is a structural or mechanical problem with the hardware such as a loose screw or broken rod
- You have pain or some other problem directly associated with the hardware, such as painful prominence of the hardware against the skin, an allergic reaction to nickel, or an infection around the hardware

The surgery to remove the hardware is not trivial. Like any surgery, it involves risks. Hardware removal should be considered a last resort to solving a hardware-induced problem.

What Does the Hardware Feel Like?

The amount of hardware installed in your body during scoliosis surgery can be extensive. Many patients wonder how this will feel. People who have undergone the surgery give varied answers on this issue. The hardware itself does not actually touch any nerve endings, so you should not feel it directly.

Some of the hardware attaches to nothing but other hardware—the rods attach to screws or hooks, and the cross-links attach to the rods, for instance.

What you may feel, however, is some of the hardware pressing against the inside of your skin or on other muscles. This is more common if you are slim or have a small build, or if you have a posterior-approach surgery, in which case the rods and other hardware will be positioned outwards. This may be noticeable when leaning against a chair back, for example. I know from my experience that sitting in certain chairs causes me to sit at just such an angle that I feel pressure at the lower cross-link that bridges my two rods. I would not describe this as painful, but it can be irritating enough to cause me to reposition myself.

The extent to which the hardware can be felt or observed also depends on the area of vertebrae fused. The spine is not equidistant from the surface of the skin at all locations. The cervical vertebrae, for instance, are closer to the surface of the skin than the lumbar vertebrae. Therefore, instrumentation in the cervical region may be more prominent and thus potentially more noticeable than instrumentation in the thoracic or lumbar regions.

Your surgeon will make every effort to minimize the prominence of the hardware he or she installs. However, as mentioned in the previous section, if the hardware causes severe irritation it can be removed once your fusion solidifies.

Frequently-Asked Questions

Q) Will the instrumentation ever rust?
A) No, neither stainless steel nor titanium instrumentation will ever rust.

Q) Will the instruments set off metal detector alarms at security checkpoints?
A) The vast majority of surgeons will answer no, and I do not personally know anyone whose instrumentation has set off a metal detector. However, I have heard a few individuals claim that their hardware sets off some detectors. Normally instrumentation is buried so deeply under bone and tissue that a metal detector's field cannot penetrate it. It is possible that very thin patients with instrumentation placed close to the surface of their skin may not have enough of a buffer to escape detection. It is also possible that some de-

tectors are simply more sensitive than others. Another explanation is that some detectors are not sensitive to the specific alloys used in most spinal instrumentation. If this issue ever becomes a problem for you, your doctor can give you a card to carry that identifies you as having metal implants.

Q) How much does the instrumentation weigh?
A) Most patients will carry an extra one to three pounds of weight. You will not notice it.

Common Surgical Complications

Most people who undergo scoliosis surgery do not encounter complications. Do not let the term "complications" scare you. A complication is anything that occurs during or after surgery that deviates from the textbook-perfect case. Most complications associated with scoliosis surgery are not serious, in the sense that they are not life threatening, and they are correctable. While you should not refuse to have surgery because of these risks, you should at least be familiar with what they are and discuss any that particularly concern you with your surgeon.

Infections. The body is susceptible to infections any time an incision is made. Urinary tract infections caused by the Foley catheter postoperatively are also possible. Infections are usually treated effectively with antibiotics and occur in less than 5% of scoliosis surgery cases. If a severe infection develops postoperatively around the incision site or the instrumentation, a second surgery may be necessary to clean out the infected area, and in some cases the hardware must be removed.

Pneumothorax. Scoliosis surgeons operate in close proximity to the lungs, which may inadvertently be punctured by a surgeon's tool, a piece of instrumentation, or a cut bone. A pneumothorax occurs when air is trapped between the lung and the chest wall. The air can either come from inside the lung or from outside the chest cavity. As air builds up in this space, the pressure against the lung can cause it to collapse. In a controlled hospital setting, re-inflating a lung is not particularly difficult. Pneumothoraxes may also seal themselves fairly quickly.

Drug reactions. Some people are allergic to the various anesthetics, painkillers, and antibiotics given to patients during surgery and recovery. These reactions are rarely life threatening, and drug substitutes are almost always available.

Pneumonia. During recovery, you will be on your back for extended periods and fluid will slowly accumulate in your lungs. If the fluid buildup reaches too high a level, pneumonia can develop. To prevent this, nursing staff will encourage you to cough frequently to clear your lungs. This can hurt while you are healing but is important preventive maintenance. Exercising your lungs using an *inspirometer* (see Chapter 6) before and after surgery can also help prevent pneumonia.

Neurological damage. Any time a surgeon operates close to the spine, there is always a chance of injuring the spinal cord. This is extremely rare, occurring in far less than 1% of all scoliosis surgeries. Injuries to the spinal cord could result in paralysis, sensory and motor deficiencies, pain, numbness, tingling, and other potentially serious conditions. Some effects are temporary. Some patients, for example, lose all feeling in their legs postperatively for a week and then suddenly regain sensation.

To minimize the risk of damaging the spinal cord, during surgery the nerves in the spinal cord are continuously monitored electronically. If there is any doubt that the readings from the monitors are reliable, surgeons will perform a *wake-up test* to check your motor function in the most direct way possible: by waking you up for a few minutes *during* surgery and asking you to wiggle your toes. This sounds horrifying, but during this time your pain will continue to be controlled. After surgery, few patients remember waking up.

Longer-Term Surgical Risks and Complications

While most patients will have one surgery and never again need treatment for their scoliosis, complications can arise later in life that require surgical correction. Today, this is called *revision surgery,* although it was once referred to by the more grim-sounding term, *salvage surgery*. In general, revision surgery is necessary in five situations:

1. The fusion fails (pseudarthrosis) or the instrumentation breaks or comes loose
2. The curvature progresses above and/or below the fused section
3. Severe postural problems develop (flatback)
4. The intervertebral discs above and/or below the fusion become damaged or degenerated, or
5. One side of a child's spine continues to grow (crankshafting)

These cases are examined below.

Pseudarthrosis and instrumentation breakage. Pseudarthrosis is the failure of the vertebrae to fuse successfully. This has two detrimental effects, both of which are related. First, without a successful fusion, the curvature will not be corrected and may continue to progress. Second, without a successful fusion, the instrumentation will lack a solid foundation on which to attach. For instance, a lone unfused vertebra may move freely just enough to prevent a pedicle screw from being securely held. If the pedicle screw loses its anchor, the rod attached to the screw may become unstable.

It is difficult to say how many scoliosis surgery patients develop pseudarthrosis. The statistics vary widely from 5-30%, though the rate is dropping over time due to better surgical techniques. A 2005 study of 96 adult patients revealed that 17% experienced pseudarthrosis.[9] The study also found that patients older than 55 years and those with fusions of more than twelve vertebrae were at increased risk for pseudarthrosis. Pseudarthrosis occurs less frequently in children and adolescents than in adults.

One reason for the lack of a good statistic is that many cases of pseudarthrosis are never detected. In fact, there is no reliable way to verify whether a fusion is solid or has failed. Conventional x-rays and more sophisticated imaging systems like CAT (computerized axial tomography) scans and MRIs (magnetic resonance imaging systems) may not reveal the state of the fusion. Even opening up a patient and inspecting the spine directly may not provide a definitive answer.

Unfortunately, the way most cases of pseudarthrosis are detected is by instrumentation breakage (called *failure*). Patients usually become aware, quickly and painfully, when instrumentation breaks. The pain from dislodged metal hardware poking into one's back muscles or skin can be excruciating. In some cases, though, patients are not aware there is a problem for years—and sometimes they will never notice one.

Many things can cause pseudarthrosis. In rare cases, it is the result of improper placement or usage of the instrumentation by the surgeon, or insufficient bone grafting. The instrumentation may also be broken by excessive force to the spine after surgery, such as from a severe accident. And sometimes, well, these things just happen.

If you develop pseudarthrosis or if your instrumentation fails for any reason, you may need revision surgery to re-fuse the involved vertebrae and/or re-attach the existing hardware, or new hardware may be installed at this time.

The great news is that pseudarthrosis in new scoliosis surgery cases is becoming increasingly rare. Successful fusion rates are much higher today than in previous years due to better instrumentation and better surgical techniques. Patients with the now obsolete Harrington rods have far higher rates of pseudarthrosis and instrumentation breakage than patients with the new segmental systems.

Decompensation. After a spinal fusion, an unfused portion of the spine directly above or below the fused section may begin to curve, or a compensatory curve that existed preoperatively may fail to straighten on its own. These situations can lead to an imbalance in which the remaining structural curvature that was surgically corrected is not counter-balanced by the newly-developing curve or old compensatory curves. If this imbalance, called decompensation, is severe, additional surgery may be necessary to extend the section originally fused and instrumented to encompass the newly-problematic section.

Decompensation most commonly occurs as a result of selective fusions in which only the structural components of a spine were fused and instrumented, in the hope that all compensatory curves would correct on their own (they usually do, but not always). Decompensation may also occur if the spine was fused and instrumented in an already unbalanced position.

Flatback. Flatback (also called *flatback syndrome* or *fixed sagittal imbalance*) is the progressive loss of the normal sagittal curve in the lumbar region. A normal lower back curves gently inward (lordosis). In flatback syndrome, the patient's lower back does not curve at all—it appears flat. Over time, the affected individual will begin to lean forward perpetually and will have trouble standing upright without bending the knees. This, in turn, weakens back muscles and causes pain and fatigue. The condition may worsen over time because the increased stress placed on the lumbar region tends to cause the discs to degenerate.

Flatback is caused by instrumentation in the lumbar region that pushes too hard on the vertebrae to which it is attached. This condition is not uncommon among those who had Harrington rods implanted. These rods, unlike modern segmental instrumentation, applied excessive forces on the spine to straighten it. While this resulted in drastically reduced curvatures, it also tended to flatten normal lordosis. Fortunately, new cases of flatback syndrome are far less common today due to better instrumentation, better surgeon training, and refined surgical techniques. Flatback is seen in only about 1% of modern surgeries.

Most cases of flatback syndrome are not serious enough to warrant revision surgery. If revision surgery proves necessary, however, the surgeon must first undo the previous procedure by removing the old hardware and then perform one or more *osteotomies.* An osteotomy is the resecting (cutting) of a vertebra so that it can then be fused (or re-fused) in a position that restores normal lordosis. The surgeon will typically implant new instrumentation using a combined anterior/posterior approach. The surgeon may also remove discs between the lumbar vertebrae and in their place insert large grafts of bone or small metal cages filled with tiny pieces of bone to promote fusion.

Disc degeneration. All the discs between vertebrae naturally become weaker over time. The discs in a fused area of spine, however, do not degenerate. To compensate, the discs in regions above or below the fused section will thus take more of a beating and degenerate faster. This can lead to severe pain around the degenerated discs. Surgery to correct this problem will usually involve removing the degenerated discs and fusing or re-fusing the involved vertebrae.

Crankshafting. If the spine of a young child who is not yet skeletally mature is fused only from the back (posteriorly), the front (anterior) vertebrae can continue to grow and deform in a twisting "corkscrew" manner during the child's growth spurt. This can be prevented by performing a combined anterior/posterior (A/P) spinal fusion. If this was not done, however, and crankshaft develops, complex revision surgery will be necessary.

Bracing Failure—Why do I Need Surgery Now?

Many older individuals who wore a brace in their adolescent years are now confronting the prospect of impending scoliosis surgery. If this describes your situation, you may be wondering why this is the case. You were probably told when you were first given the brace that wearing it would prevent you from ever needing surgery. This turned out to be true in the majority of cases.

However, we now know that bracing does not always work. The statistics vary based on a variety of factors, but several studies performed in the 1990s indicate that as many as 20-40% of patients who were braced in their adolescent years will still require surgery at some point in their life. Why this happens is not well understood. Several factors seem to contribute to success or failure rates:

Patient diligence. Patients who wore their brace diligently are less likely to require surgery. Most adolescents do not wear their braces as much as instructed by their orthopedists. For those who did, as few as 10% will require surgery later in life.

Number of hours per day the brace is worn. Some orthopedists do not ask patients to wear a brace full-time. Research suggests a direct correlation between how many hours per day one wears a brace with the likelihood of needing surgery later. Patients who wore their brace twenty-three hours per day tend to need surgery less often than those who were told to wear it only a few hours per day.

Severity of curvature at the time bracing treatment began. Patients who began wearing a brace when their curve was below 30° tend to need surgery less often than those who began a bracing treatment when their curves were more advanced.

Number of months the brace is worn. Bracing works best when the brace is worn until a patient is skeletally mature. Some orthopedists, however, allow patients to stop wearing their brace before this point is reached.

Type of brace. Patients who wore what is called a Charleston Bending Brace (sometimes just called a nighttime brace, because it is typically only worn at night) tend to need surgery more frequently than those who wore Boston or Milwaukee Braces. In some cases, orthopedists prescribed the wrong brace for the patient's curve. Boston Braces are only effective at holding curves with an apex below the T9 vertebra (lumbar curves and some thoracic and thoracolumbar curves), while Milwaukee Braces are required to hold curves with an apex higher in the back (most thoracic curves).

Quality of brace construction. Braces are custom-fitted to every patient. Nonetheless, there is some art in crafting a brace correctly. Braces that did not fit well may not have worked at all.

Despite these contributing factors, sometimes the reason for bracing failure in a particular case remains unknown. I wore a Milwaukee Brace diligently, twenty-three hours a day for two years until my bones stopped growing. The brace seemed to work; my curve was stable for the two years I wore the brace. Even so, after I stopped wearing it, my curve slowly began to increase and I ultimately needed surgery. These situations are tragic but are a reality of scoliosis.

Do not take this to mean that bracing has no merit. On the contrary, bracing has been proven to be effective in arresting the progression of *most* cases of adolescent idiopathic scoliosis in which the curve is between 25° and 40°. This alone, in my view, is sufficient reason for adolescents to try bracing if an orthopedist says it is a viable treatment option. Ensuring that the right brace is prescribed, that it is properly made, that it is worn diligently full-time, and that it is worn for a sufficient time period should help increase the likelihood that one will never need surgery.

Scoliosis Surgery for Infants and Juveniles

Scoliosis surgery is generally not indicated for very young children. This is because, unlike an adult, the spines of young children are continuing to grow. Fusing the spine of a child who has not reached skeletal maturity would restrict his or her natural growth. This has to be balanced, however, with the reality that the curves of some young children progress at such a rapid rate that failure to intervene surgically could prove life threatening. Orthopedic surgeons thus have three options.

One option is to implant a type of instrumentation called a growing rod. This kind of rod is essentially an internal brace. It stabilizes the spine to provide partial correction and arrest curve progression. The rods are adjustable; the surgeon will perform follow-up surgeries about every six to nine months until the child reaches adolescence in order to expand the rods to accommodate the child's growth. In this approach, spinal fusion is not performed until adolescence.

The key advantage of this approach is that the child's spine is allowed to attain its optimal length prior to fusion. This will allow the child to ultimately be closer to—though not quite reach—his or her genetically-programmed height. The obvious downside to this approach is the distressing number of surgeries the child must endure—as many as two per year for up to ten (or more!) years. Repeat surgeries cause pain and psychological trauma, and present the usual roster of surgical risks. Fortunately, children tend to recover from these adjustment surgeries fairly quickly.

The second option is to perform a surgery like those done on adults. This usually alleviates the need for any further surgeries, but has an unpleasant downside: the fused portion of the child's spine will never grow, thus the child will never reach his or her full height potential. If the child is already near his or her maximum height, a conventional fusion and instrumentation procedure may be acceptable in exchange for a few inches of height.

The third option is called a *short segment apical fusion*. In this approach, only a small number of vertebrae at the apex (the "peak") of the curve are fused.

This permanently corrects and stabilizes the most deformed section of the curve. However, a more extensive long fusion will still need to be performed once the child reaches adolescence.

Clearly, none of these options is ideal. To maximize the chances of a successful procedure, parents of young children with scoliosis should consult an orthopedist who specializes in infantile or juvenile scoliosis.

Deciding to Have Surgery

Making the decision to have surgery is not easy. Even if the rationale for having surgery is clear, surgery can be a frightening prospect. Here are a few suggestions to assist in the decision-making process.

Take advantage of the fact that time is on your side. Scoliosis surgery is almost never urgent. Unless you are in unbearable pain or your heart and lungs are being dangerously compressed due to your curvature, you do not need to have surgery right now. You can take as much time as you need to research scoliosis thoroughly and talk to others who have been through the surgery.

Although holding off on having surgery is always an option, there are consequences for waiting too long. In general, the younger you are, the faster you will recover, the greater the correction possible, and the lower the chances of serious surgical complications. On the other hand, surgical procedures may continue to improve as they have over the last twenty years, thus offering improved correction, faster recovery with less pain, and fewer complications should you decide to delay surgery. Only you, in consultation with your orthopedist and with those who care about you, can make the right decision.

Get additional medical opinions. Every orthopedic surgeon is different. Based on his or her specialization and experience, each surgeon may give you a different assessment of whether you are a strong surgical candidate, how he or she would approach your surgery, and what level of correction may be achieved. See *Choosing a Surgical Team* in Chapter 4.

Involve others in your decision. It is useful to gain perspective from those you trust. Discuss your condition and your surgeon's prognosis with your family, friends, and others who are important to you and whose opinions you value. Talking it out and getting feedback will give you more confidence that you are making the right decision, whatever that may be.

A word of caution: be certain that the people you talk to are not grossly misinformed about scoliosis, nor have financial or other interests in recommending alternative treatments that are not clinically proven to be of benefit.

Make sure that you are being realistic about your expectations from surgery and are willing to accept some risks. As mentioned earlier, no surgeon can predict with certainty how much your curvature can be corrected or how much your back pain, if you are experiencing any, can be relieved. There are no guarantees that this surgery will relieve any pain you are experiencing. It may, in fact, cause *additional* pain, or it may simply change the nature or location of your pain.

Ask your doctor to be forthcoming about all potential surgical complications. Most scoliosis surgery patients have relatively minor complications, or none whatsoever. Nonetheless, to make a well-informed decision about whether to have surgery, you need to be aware of all the complications that you may experience, however unlikely they may be. Many orthopedists will not discuss the less likely complications with you unless you bring up the subject.

CHAPTER THREE

Alternatives to Surgery

If you meet the criteria defined in Chapter 2 for being a good surgical candidate, surgery is, regrettably, the only viable option to correct your curvature and halt its progression. The only other recourse is to attempt to control the pain, discomfort, stiffness, and soreness often associated with scoliosis. This approach—pain management—addresses the symptoms but ignores the underlying cause. It can buy you time, but if your curvature is already severe or progressing rapidly, surgery will almost certainly be necessary eventually. The most common methods of scoliosis pain management are described in this chapter.

Medications

There are several types of medication that can control the pain caused by a moderate to severe curvature:

Over-the-counter analgesics (painkillers) and anti-inflammatories, such as acetaminophen (Tylenol®), ibuprofen (Advil®, Motrin®), naproxen (Aleve®), or aspirin may be sufficient to control your pain. You should never exceed the recommended dosages of these medications. You should also be aware that these medications may have side effects, especially in combination with other drugs. Long-term use of acetaminophen, for example, can damage your liver, especially if you drink excessive amounts of alcohol. These drugs can also cause problems for those who have gastrointestinal problems such as ulcers.

Prescription-strength painkillers, such as hydrocodone. If over-the-counter painkillers do not work for you, speak to your doctor about trying prescription-strength narcotics or anti-inflammatories. These medicines relieve pain effectively for most people but may have serious and dangerous side effects, commonly including fatigue and dizziness, which render them poor choices for daily or long-term use. They can also be addictive. Some find that higher doses of over-the-counter pain medications are just as effective at controlling pain as these narcotics, and certainly carry fewer side effects. See *Pain Control Medications* for more information.

Over-the-counter and prescription muscle relaxants. These medications relax the muscles that are often tensed by scoliotic curves. Unfortunately, these medications can also make you profoundly tired and thus prevent you from driving or performing any other tasks that require acute mental focus.

Over-the-counter medicated creams and patches (Icy Hot®, BENGAY®). The active ingredients in these creams and patches—methyl salicylate and/or menthol—provide some pain relief by masking muscle pain with a warm, tingly sensation. They are not muscle relaxants, per se, but they can help relieve muscle tension. Because these are applied *topically* (at the location of pain), the medicine contained in the cream does not circulate through your entire body and thus has no side effects. These products have a few minor disadvantages: they tend to be shorter-acting than orally-taken medications, they emit a strong odor which some find unpleasant and which can irritate the eyes, they leave a slightly greasy residue on your hands and wherever applied, and they can only be applied where you can reach (unless someone is applying it for you).

Simple Pain Management Techniques

In addition to, or in lieu of, medications, you may want to try some common, simple techniques for minimizing pain.

Exercise. Exercise really should not be viewed as an *alternative* to surgery. Rather, it becomes even more important if you are going to have surgery. For scoliosis patients in particular, certain exercises can help relieve the pain associated with the curvature. I would recommend you obtain the professional advice of a physical therapist or personal trainer to identify the specific exercises that would most benefit you. In general, these will be anything that strengthens and increases the flexibility of the muscles in your back, shoulders, and abdomen. You should consult a doctor before beginning an exercise program.

Relaxation techniques. A relaxed mind and body can diminish the perception of pain. There are a variety of methods to help you relax, all of which are free, take minimal time out of your day, and can be done anytime, anywhere. It is beyond the scope of this book to explore all of these techniques, but briefly, they include controlled breathing, progressive muscle relaxation, and meditation. There are plenty of good books to help you develop these techniques. There are also professional experts and courses on stress management that cover the same material. Whether you have surgery or not, these are good practices to adopt for managing both pain and stress.

Get a better bed. Whether standing or laying down, your back is most relaxed when your spine is in its natural position—straight. Of course, if you have scoliosis your spine is never straight. But sleeping on an unsupportive bed can place your scoliotic curvature in an even more incorrectly curved position for the eight or so hours a night that an average person sleeps. In addition to a poor night's sleep, this can lead to muscle fatigue that interferes with your daily activities.

The optimal mattress is the one that best helps you maintain a *relatively* straight posture (keeps your spine as aligned as possible), and that you find the most comfortable. Many mattress manufacturers make claims that their beds are "orthopedic," but there is no universal definition of what this means.

A proper sleeping position is also important. Sleeping on your side, with the knees bent or with a pillow between the knees is the best way to maintain proper body posture. If you must sleep on your back, place a pillow under your knees to support the normal curve of the lower back.

Sleeping on your stomach or with your head elevated on an oversized pillow arches the natural curves of the back, as well as increases pressure on the diaphragm and lungs. These positions can lead to restless tossing and turning and therefore a less refreshing sleep.

Heat and cold. Heat is a wonderful muscular pain reliever. Heat promotes blood circulation in the area to which it is applied. Hot showers, hot tubs, steam rooms, hot water bottles, and heating pads are all effective yet temporary means of pain management. Cold treatments (also called *cryotherapy*) in the form of cold packs or ice massage can be effective, too.

Professional Pain Management

If your pain is infringing on the quality of your life and you have tried the simpler, more conservative pain management remedies like exercise and non-prescription medication, you may want to consult a professional pain specialist or physical therapist.

Pain specialists. Most pain specialists are medical doctors who have specific training in pain management. Many pain specialists are trained or concurrently practice as anesthesiologists. Be sure to evaluate the specialist's credentials, because some self-professed pain specialists are not, in fact, medical doctors and primarily advocate the kinds of alternative treatments described in the Quackery section later in this chapter.

A pain specialist may order a series of tests to determine precisely what is causing your pain. Based on test results, he or she may then recommend a wide spectrum of solutions. This may include many of the treatment methods described previously, ranging from non-prescription and prescription medications to special exercises or physical therapy. Also included may be more extreme treatments such as nerve blocks, tiny machines placed inside your body that automatically deliver pain medication, electrical stimulation therapies, or the deliberate destruction of nerves that are carrying pain signals to your brain.

For severe, chronic pain management, a pain specialist may prescribe the use of a TENS unit. TENS stands for Transcutaneous Electrical Nerve Stimulation. These devices deliver a painless electrical current *transcutaneously* (through your skin, via electrode patches) to certain nerves that relay pain signals. The small amount of heat generated by these electrical signals relieves pain for most people, but success rates vary tremendously. TENS units can either be stationary or portable. You may need to visit the office of a pain specialist or physical therapist for treatment, or you may be able to get a portable unit for home use.

To find a pain specialist, ask for a referral from your primary care physician or orthopedist, or consult your health insurance provider. Many insurance providers have a list of doctors in their network under a category called "pain management," though some may combine these listings under "anesthesiology." Unlike other pain management techniques such as chiropractic or massage therapy, insurance providers will usually cover fees from a pain specialist if there is a clear need to consult one.

Physical therapy. For an individual with scoliosis, the goal of physical therapy is to relieve pain and restore normal body function and movement, if limited. A physical therapist would do this in a several ways. First, the therapist would educate the patient on ways to avoid pain by practicing good posture whether sitting, standing, or laying down, as well as by practicing good techniques for bending and lifting. Failure to follow such techniques may exacerbate pain. For example, sitting hunched over a computer keyboard for too long can cause back or shoulder pain, so the therapist would teach you how to find a better chair and to sit in a position that reduces the stresses that cause the pain.

Second, the therapist would focus on strength and flexibility training through an array of exercises. Some of these exercises would be conducted at the therapist's facility, while you would do some at home. In particular, the trunk muscles, the abdominals, spine extensors, and legs should be strengthened. Leg strengthening is important so that you can properly lift objects from the floor using your leg muscles rather than those of your back.

Finally, the therapist may employ technological or other approaches to treating the pain directly, such as electrical stimulation, ultrasound, or massage therapy.

Most health insurance plans will pay for physical therapy if you have a referral from a doctor.

Alternative Treatments

In addition to medications and simple pain management techniques, there are several alternative treatment programs available. All of these are more expensive and more time-consuming than the options listed above. Whether they are of any tangible benefit is hotly debated and clearly subjective.

Beyond minimizing the pain associated with scoliosis, some will argue that these techniques can also actually correct a scoliotic curvature or halt its progression. Such claims are completely unsubstantiated. The only way to permanently correct a scoliotic curve is surgically. None of the treatments described in this section have been proven to reduce a curvature or stop the progression of a curve, and all of these treatments provide only temporary relief from pain. In addition, pursuing these treatments in lieu of bracing a growing child who is a suitable candidate for this treatment means that you may miss a narrow window of opportunity to halt a progressive curve at an early stage.

Chiropractic. Most people intuitively think of chiropractors as "back doctors," and thus there is a natural tendency to seek help from a chiropractor before visiting an orthopedic surgeon or contemplating spine surgery. Make no mistake, though: chiropractors have not received the level of training in orthopedics that an orthopedic surgeon has, and few chiropractors are specifically trained on scoliosis. The credential of "doctor of chiropractic" (D.C.) is not at all similar to a true medical doctor (M.D.). Even so, many health insurance plans cover at least some level of chiropractic treatment.

Chiropractic care is all about forcing misaligned (what chiropractors call *subluxated*) vertebrae back into their correct position. Chiropractors use a variety of means to do this, ranging from hand thrusts (which chiropractors call *adjustments*) to traction tables and machines and electrical stimulation. Some chiropractors also practice other treatments described in this chapter, such as acupuncture, heat and cold therapy, or other modalities.

Does it help scoliosis? Some scoliosis sufferers say it has relieved their pain and claim it has arrested the progression of their curve. Others say it relieved their pain temporarily and felt good, but did not solve the underlying problem. And still others say it did not help at all. Most people would agree that a visit to a chiropractor can make your back feel better, at least temporarily.

While chiropractic care may effectively relieve your pain, you should know that there are no clinical studies to prove that chiropractic care actually reverses a curvature or arrests its progression. Intuitively, it does not seem physically possible that hand thrusts, machines that pull your spine, or tiny electrically-induced contractions in the muscles around your spine can permanently re-align your vertebrae. And many chiropractors would agree with that. In fact, a 2001 study of children with minor scoliotic curvatures provided some evidence that chiropractic care has, as the researchers observed, "no discernable effect on the severity of the curves as a function of age, curve severity, frequency of care or attending physician."[10] Forty-two 6- to 12-year olds with curves ranging from 6-20° were given chiropractic adjustments, heel-lifts, and "postural/lifestyle counseling" for one year. The researchers' conclusion: "Full-spine chiropractic adjustments with heel-lifts and postural/lifestyle counseling are not effective in reducing the severity of scoliotic curves." Ironically, both the researchers who conducted the study were themselves chiropractors.

Network chiropractic. Unlike traditional chiropractic, which focuses on the vertebrae, network chiropractic focuses on the spinal cord. Network chiropractors argue that all of the body's self-healing capabilities rely on the health of the spinal cord. If the spinal cord—which contains the primary nerves in the human body—is compressed, they argue, one will feel pain and could suffer from a host of ailments, including scoliosis.

While compressed nerves can certainly cause pain, it is unclear how network chiropractors resolve the compression. Unlike traditional chiropractic or massage therapy, both of which involve direct physical manipulation of bones or muscles, the mechanism by which network chiropractic reduces pain or actually corrects a spinal curvature defies logic. Network chiropractors employ a very light touch to the spine that allegedly stimulates the spinal cord. For someone with scoliosis, this stimulation supposedly focuses the patient's brain on the curved region of the spine and encourages the body to correct the deformity. No clinical study supports this. Despite the absence of a logical rationale behind how network chiropractic works, some people with scoliosis feel it helps.

Massage therapy. A curved spine causes the muscles in your shoulders and around your spine to misalign or become stretched or compressed. This, in turn, causes uncomfortable tension or spasms. A massage therapist can relieve this tension not only in your back, but also in all the muscle groups throughout your body that can be directly or indirectly affected by your spinal deformity. As almost everyone knows, a good massage just feels great.

Like chiropractic treatments, the relief achievable through massage therapy is temporary. Your back may feel relaxed and pain-free for several hours or even a day or two, but the discomfort will return as the effects of gravity once again tense your muscles.

You should try to find a massage therapist experienced or familiar with spine problems. You should also seek someone who is licensed by the state in which you live as an RMT (registered massage therapist). When you first visit with a massage therapist, you should inform him or her about your scoliosis and the nature of the pain you are feeling.

If you want to see a massage therapist *after* you have scoliosis surgery, wait until the soreness and any pain related to the surgery has subsided. You should also inform the therapist of precisely where and what hardware has been installed in your back. You *can* be hurt if a therapist puts too much pressure on or near the hardware.

Some schools that train massage therapists offer "student massages" at reduced prices, though if your curvature is severe I would advise against seeing someone without more experience.

Rolfing. Rolfing® (named after Dr. Ida Rolf, who invented the technique) is a cross between chiropractic care and deep tissue massage. Unlike a chiropractor, who uses hand thrusts to re-align bones, "rolfers" make milder manipulations with their hands and elbows to stimulate the soft connective tissues that surround the bones; they do not move the bone itself. In this sense rolfing is more like massage. Unlike massage therapists, though, rolfers claim that they can finely separate tissue layers that are stuck together and can re-align muscles that have been knocked out of their correct position.

Many rolfing patients have been in accidents in which certain regions of their bodies have been forcibly misaligned through trauma. For such cases, rolfers claim they can restore normal bone positions. Rolfers concede that they cannot straighten bones that are structurally deformed, as are the vertebrae in some scoliotic patients. Nonetheless, rolfers argue that they can help scoliosis patients by restoring the pulled or compressed soft tissues surrounding the spine to their normal state.

Two points about rolfing in comparison to chiropractic care or massage therapy are worth noting. First, like massage therapy, rolfing more directly addresses the pain that often accompanies scoliosis rather than the bone deformity itself. Rolfers work on muscles, not on bones. Second, rolfers typically know more about bone deformities than massage therapists. This is because many people who see rolfers are victims of trauma or other types of accidents; rolfers are thus trained to treat those with bone deformities.

Pilates®. Created by Joseph Pilates in the 1920s, the Pilates Method is an exercise program focused on improving flexibility and strength throughout the body. Participants perform a series of controlled movements on floor mats and on specially-designed equipment that somewhat resemble resistance training machines found in gyms and physical therapy clinics. Compared to traditional resistance training workouts, participants perform relatively few repetitions of each movement, focusing more on precision and proper form than on the quantity of work performed. As such, Pilates is not an aerobic workout, and it does not build significant muscle mass nor burn much fat. Workouts are usually supervised by an instructor on a one-on-one basis or conducted in small groups.

The alleged benefits of Pilates for someone with scoliosis include strengthening of the support muscles in the abdomen and around the spine (particularly in the lower back), reducing muscle tension, increasing the flexibility of bones and joints, and improving posture. A nice facet of Pilates is that each workout is tailored to your specific abilities and goals and is supervised by a trained instructor. This may be safer than walking into a gym on your own and trying resistance training equipment. In addition, many Pilates studios now offer other complementary services described in this chapter, such as massage therapy, chiropractic care, and physical therapy.

Acupuncture and acupressure. Both acupuncture and acupressure are healing techniques based on a belief that energy travels throughout one's body along meridians, or channels. The Chinese are said to have mapped out these channels thousands of years ago. If the energy circulating through any of these channels is disrupted, as allegedly happens with a crooked spine, pain can result. These points of disruption allegedly must be stimulated to restore the normal flow of energy. This stimulation can be in the form of placing small needles into the skin at these points (acupuncture), or by applying gentle pressure with one's fingers (acupressure). Acupressure adds a bit of a massage component to treatment.

That much is the theory. Western medicine has not confirmed the existence of these energy channels. Even Chinese medical schools that research the mechanics of how acupuncture and acupressure may work have not uncovered a scientific explanation. Despite any understanding of how or why it may work, some people claim that it has cured them of chronic pain and chronic disorders ranging from allergies to depression. Others claim it has done nothing. Acupuncturists readily admit that acupuncture will not restore a spine to a straight position. They do profess, however, that it can temporarily diminish or eliminate pain caused by a scoliotic curvature.

Most people undergoing acupuncture treatment visit an acupuncturist once a week. The number of visits required to experience any benefit varies by person and by the nature and degree of pain. And, again, some people will never experience any improvement. Others claim that they experienced significant pain reduction on their first visit. Each visit typically lasts up to one hour. In each visit, as many as twenty needles are placed in the back to reduce pain in the muscles surrounding the spine. Additional needles may be placed at other points throughout the body to help alleviate pain or other problems tangentially caused by scoliosis, such as headaches or pain in the hips.

Interestingly, Chinese natives who were educated in acupuncture in China often hold the U.S. equivalent of a medical degree. You may find that Chinese acupuncturists practicing in the U.S. have an impressive level of knowledge about scoliosis and orthopedics in general. By contrast, virtually anyone can become a licensed acupuncturist in the U.S. without any medical background whatsoever.

Yoga. Yoga is an ancient discipline that combines various postures, stretching, and breathing and relaxation techniques. Yoga—which is practiced in a variety of forms today—can benefit anyone suffering from scoliosis in several ways. First, yoga stretches the spine. This releases tension in the muscles of the back that surround the spine, thereby reducing the pain associated with scoliosis. Certain yoga poses also help strengthen the muscles of the abdomen and back, which can also reduce pain and promote better posture. This is not to say that yoga actually corrects scoliotic curves. However, yoga can help "train" individuals to maintain the best posture they can, which combats the perception, if not the reality, that the individual is not properly aligned. For individuals who lean to one side due to their curvature, yoga may help them achieve a more natural stance and better balance when walking or standing. Another critical benefit of yoga is that it is relaxing. Relaxation can help reduce the pain, stress, and anxiety that often accompanies scoliosis.

Some patients claim that practicing yoga diligently has reduced or even eliminated their scoliosis. This has not been substantiated by clinical studies. It may be true, however, that yoga can temporarily reduce scoliotic curves a small amount by both lengthening the spine and building-up the abdominal and back muscles that support it.

Not everyone with scoliosis will find that they are able to perform yoga. Individuals with more severe cases of scoliosis simply may not be able to achieve some of the yoga poses. As with any exercise program of this type, you should consult your doctor before beginning yoga.

Quackery

Scoliosis surgery is such a terrifying prospect for some that they will embrace any form of treatment to avoid it. Regrettably, far too many people and organizations prey on the fears and hopes of scoliosis sufferers, offering them "solutions" which have no demonstrated clinical viability. Many of these programs combine elements of chiropractic care, massage, exercises, and special diets. Some programs add bracing, vibration therapy (which is exactly what it sounds like), and even the placing of magnets or oils on the back.

There are so many "treatment programs" propagating on the Internet today that it would be impossible to list them all. Two of them are worth noting, however. The first one, from the Copes Foundation, is arguably the best known and most popular alternative scoliosis treatment program, and the second one, raindrop therapy, is mentioned because it effectively illustrates just how bizarre alternative therapy claims can be.

The Copes Foundation (www.scoliosis.com) currently markets a program that it claims corrects scoliotic curves without surgery. This program, called the Scoliosis Treatment Recovery System (STRS), combines wearing a brace up to twenty hours a day with frequent visits to a chiropractor, electrical muscle stimulation, daily exercise routines, a special diet, vitamin and hormone supplements, and frequent chemical analyses. Participants in this program are told that they must continue this program for years, if not the rest of their life.

STRS sounds appealing in that it is a non-surgical approach that promises correction, not just stabilization of the curve, and in that it treats the whole individual with special diets and exercises. Unfortunately, there is no clinical data to support that STRS actually works. Patient testimonials suggest that STRS can result in some degree of *temporary* correction, but the curve will relapse to its original severity level if the program is stopped. In my opinion, this alone should be reason not to bother with STRS, but there are two other good reasons. First, STRS is an incredibly time-consuming program. Patients are expected to visit a chiropractor for adjustments up to three times per week, have testing done up to four times per week, and do exercises every day—plus wear a special brace for up to twenty hours per day. Few people realistically have that much time to dedicate to the program for the rest of their lives. The other problem is that STRS is extremely expensive, costing thousands of dollars in fees per year. Insurance programs will not cover the entire STRS treatment program, though some may cover the chiropractic care portion.

Perhaps the most bizarre alternative treatment for scoliosis is called raindrop therapy, invented by a doctor who believes that scoliosis is caused by a virus or bacteria (there is no scientific evidence to support this). The pathogens allegedly irritate the spine and causes it to inflame, thus somehow knocking the spine out of alignment. The doctor's solution: drop a series of oils onto the surface of the patient's skin, which are absorbed into the spine and destroy the pathogens. Inside the oils are natural herbs like oregano, basil, marjoram, and thyme. While these may smell nice and certainly enhance the flavor of virtually any Italian dish, these ingredients do not kill viruses or bacteria, nor do they re-align a spine.

My advice is to be skeptical of any treatment that cannot be supported by a scientific study performed by reputable researchers who have no vested interest in the study's outcome. Many people touting their miracle solutions argue that media coverage of their solution somehow proves its worth. But, the media often covers alternative therapies and frequently concludes their coverage with a comment about how nothing is certain. So, trust your intuition. If it sounds too good to be true—like pouring Italian seasoning oils on your spine to correct scoliosis—it probably is.

CHAPTER FOUR

Planning Surgery

If your orthopedist deems you to be a viable surgical candidate, you will need to begin the intricate process of planning for the possibility of surgery. This chapter outlines the most important things you need to do in choosing a surgeon and hospital, determining the best time to schedule your surgery, determining how to pay for it, and establishing a support system to assist you through the potentially tough times ahead. If you decide to proceed with surgery, Chapter 5 will guide you through the preparatory steps in detail.

Before you begin this long and involved process, I recommend that you establish some kind of system to organize notes. A notebook dedicated to your surgery might be all you need, but use whatever you find most convenient. Take notes each time you visit a surgeon, talk to your insurance company, speak with other patients, attend a support group meeting, or at other times when relevant information needs to be recorded. Keep this system handy and store all your scoliosis- and surgery-related notes there.

Choosing a Surgeon

There is no magic formula for choosing the best orthopedic surgeon. As in choosing any person for any job, you need to rely on a combination of credentials, reputation, and your instinct to choose the surgeon who is best *for you*. Some surgeons are better than others in treating your specific type of curvature, your age group, and in working with your personality type. Foremost, you want a surgeon whom you trust. This person is going to operate on you and make permanent changes to your spine. If you have any doubts of his or her abilities, walk away.

Be aware that finding a scoliosis surgeon outside of a major metropolitan area can be difficult. Even if you do live in a city with several surgeons to choose from, you may want to travel elsewhere to find a surgeon you prefer. Some insurance plans will allow you to do this, but may pay reduced benefits for medical care outside their local network.

Narrowing Your Options

Your health insurance carrier may limit how many surgeons you can choose from. Below are some suggestions for finding a doctor in your area who specializes in scoliosis:

- *Ask your primary care physician.* Most physicians will know a local scoliosis surgeon, or know how to find one. If your insurance plan is an HMO that requires a physician referral to a specialist, you will need to consult your physician, regardless. It is always a good idea to keep your physician informed of your medical conditions, especially if you are considering major surgery.

- *Look under "orthopedic surgery" in your insurance carrier's medical provider directory.* This will probably not indicate a specialization in scoliosis, so you may need to call the office of each provider listed to inquire if that provider specializes in scoliosis or knows a surgeon in your area who does.

- *Contact the Scoliosis Research Society (SRS).* The SRS does not recommend or refer patients to specific scoliosis surgeons, but it does maintain a directory of orthopedic spine specialists who are SRS members. The directory is available on the SRS' website (www.srs.org), or call (414) 289-9107. Note that these records are not always up to date.

- *Search Internet discussion groups on scoliosis.* Search the archives for surgeons in your area, or post a question to the other group members asking for recommendations. A particularly good resource is the forum maintained by the National Scoliosis Foundation, at www.scoliosis.org.

- *Contact a local support group.* These can be invaluable not only in recommending specific surgeons, but also in putting you in contact with patients who have undergone surgery with local surgeons. You can find a scoliosis support group in your area that is affiliated with the Scoliosis Association by calling (800) 800-0669, or visit its website at www.scoliosis-assoc.org.

Surgeon Credentials

Credentials are important. You should seek a surgeon who has the following:

- *Board certification in orthopedic surgery by the American Academy of Orthopedic Surgeons*

- *Completion of a fellowship in spinal deformities.* This means that the surgeon has completed at least one additional year of training in spinal surgery after his or her residency in orthopedics.

- *An active membership in the Scoliosis Research Society (SRS).* The SRS is a professional organization, made up of physicians and allied health personnel. Its primary focus is on providing continuing medical education for health care professionals and on funding and supporting research in spinal deformities. Membership in the SRS indicates that at least 20% of an orthopedist's practice is in spinal deformity, that the orthopedist attends annual SRS meetings, and that he or she stays abreast of new information and new research on scoliosis. Membership in the SRS does not necessarily mean that the orthopedist is a better doctor than those who are not members of the SRS, but it does imply a commitment to the treatment of scoliosis.

- *Several years of experience in performing spinal fusions for scoliosis.* While it is possible that a newly-minted spine surgeon could perform a flawless surgery, your chances of receiving a superior operation are better with a surgeon who has several years of experience. It is difficult to state how much experience is really sufficient, but I would look for someone who has been performing spinal fusions for at least five years. Be certain that the surgeon in question has been performing spinal fusions for scoliosis cases, not other types of back surgery or spinal fusions for other disorders.

You should also understand the surgeon's specializations and experience. Most spine surgeons specialize in some combination of the following:

- One particular area of the spine (cervical, thoracic, or lumbar)
- Performing surgery on certain age groups (children versus adults)
- Using particular techniques (such as endoscopic surgery)
- First-time patient surgeries versus revision surgeries

Having a specialization does not necessarily mean that the surgeon cannot perform effective surgery on someone who falls outside his or her specialization. It usually does mean, however, that the surgeon has more training and more experience working with those groups, and thus may give you more comfort if not a better surgical outcome.

The issue of first-time surgeries versus revision surgeries is interesting. Few orthopedists claim to specialize in one over the other, and almost all orthopedists perform both types of surgeries. Nonetheless, some orthopedists perform a significantly higher percentage of revision surgeries than others, and some patients argue that certain orthopedists are just better at performing one type of surgery. There is no difference in training or any specific credentials for these two types of surgery. To find a surgeon with a better reputation for revision surgery, your best bet is to consult with local or online support groups. The national scoliosis organizations do not specifically track surgeons by this type of specialization but may have some suggestions nonetheless.

Talking to Other Patients

Ask to speak to some of the surgeon's patients who have had a surgery similar to what the surgeon recommends in your case. Ideally, try to find a patient of the same sex and of approximately the same age as you, preferably with the same type of curvature and indicated surgical approach (anterior, posterior, A/P, or endoscopic). Most patients are more than happy to share their experiences with you. These patients can usually provide you with some insight into the demeanor, personality, and attentiveness of the surgeon, both before and after surgery. They can also, of course, give you some perspectives on what the hospital stay and recovery process will be like, although this varies tremendously from patient to patient.

Communicating with Surgeons

You would of course like to feel as if you are your doctor's most important patient. But the truth is that every doctor has many patients, all of whom are important, and the time he or she can allocate to discussions with any one patient is limited. To maximize the benefits of the time you have with your surgeon, you need to do two things: be prepared and communicate efficiently.

Before you go to the surgeon's office, give some thought about exactly what you hope to accomplish from the visit. Perhaps you have a list of questions you would like to review. Or perhaps you received a second opinion and want to discuss the differences with this surgeon. Write down your expectations in your notebook. When you first meet the surgeon, tell him or her what those expectations are up-front. Whatever your goals are, do some homework before the visit. Research your questions and issues beforehand so you can better understand what your surgeon might say. Make sure that you are reasonably conversant with the terminology involved in spinal surgery.

Efficient communication with your surgeon is critical. Be clear on what you want out of your time together (remember, *you are paying for it*), but let the surgeon lead most of the conversation. Keep the conversation focused.

The first few visits to a surgeon can be overwhelming. You will be anxious, and surgeons tend to speak quickly, use medical jargon, and may bombard you with information. The effect of this is that you won't absorb everything covered in the meetings. It is therefore a good idea to bring someone with you (preferably an adult) to each meeting as a second set of ears and as a scribe.

You should focus on talking with the surgeon, while your guest should focus on listening and recording what the surgeon is saying. It would be helpful if your guest were reasonably familiar with scoliosis so he or she knows what to listen for; giving your guest this book as a primer is a good way to do that. You should also familiarize your guest beforehand with what you seek to get out of the meeting. If necessary, the guest can be useful in ensuring that everything you wanted to cover gets addressed.

Second Opinions

Before committing to surgery, you should get *at least* one other opinion from a qualified orthopedic surgeon. In addition to giving you greater confidence in your decision, this also gives you an opportunity to see the differences that exist among surgeons and to explore your full range of options. No medical professional should be offended if you inform him or her that you intend to seek a second opinion—a good doctor should actually *encourage* you to do this. If your surgeon is offended that you intend to seek another opinion, you do not want this surgeon performing surgery on you.

You should give some thought about the surgeon from whom you wish to obtain a second opinion. A good place to start is with your primary care physician. Make sure he or she understands that you need to see an orthopedic surgeon who specializes in scoliosis. You might also want to ask for recommendations from an online discussion group or a local scoliosis support group. Getting an opinion from an orthopedic center that has multiple spine surgeons on staff can be useful, as the surgeons may consult with each other if your case is unusual or particularly complex.

Another option is to purchase a second opinion on the Internet from a service such as eSpine (www.espine.com). To use this service, you simply mail in original or copies of your x-rays, complete a medical history report, and schedule a time to speak with a surgeon over the phone about your case. The cost is modest. While this may sound tempting, I do not recommend it as an alternative to getting a second opinion in person, for two reasons. First, most surgeons will not disagree about the basics of your case, such as whether you are a good candidate for surgery, whether the posterior or anterior approach is more appropriate in your case, and so on. They are more likely to disagree on the surgical specifics of how best to treat your scoliosis, such as what vertebrae to fuse or what type of instrumentation to employ. An online surgeon may give you some ideas on this, but since he or she will not be performing the actual surgery, the advice may not be as thoughtful or as relevant. More importantly, the purpose of the second opinion is as much to get a feel for the surgeon as it is to discuss your case.

When you visit the second surgeon, be sure to bring all your x-ray films (originals or copies) with you. Most offices will allow you to take your original x-ray films for evaluation by other medical professionals, as long as you return them. Other offices prefer to keep the originals but will make you copies. They may charge a modest fee for this.

Evaluating Opinions

There are six key questions you should pose to every surgeon you consult:

1. What is the magnitude (Cobb angle measurement) of my curve? This is really to double-check the Cobb angle measurement calculated by the first surgeon.
2. Which levels would you fuse, and why?
3. What surgical approach would you use, and why?
4. What is your best estimate of how much correction is achievable?
5. How many surgeries have you performed on cases similar to mine? How many have you done recently?
6. Do you foresee any unusual complications or risks in my particular case?

The chances are good that any two surgeons' opinions will vary slightly, usually more in terms of the detail of their suggested approach to performing your surgery than on the higher-level issues such as whether you are a good surgical candidate. Understand that scoliosis surgery is partly an art as well as a science. There are multiple ways to accomplish the same result, which does not necessarily mean that one approach is better than the other. Some decisions matter more than others:

- Differences in hardware choices are usually insignificant. One surgeon might want to use only pedicle screws to affix rods to your spine, while another might want to use a combination of screws and hooks. Or, one might want to use stainless steel rods while another prefers titanium. A surgeon with more experience using one type of hardware and who achieves consistently good results using it is preferable to a surgeon who waivers in his choice of instrumentation and has had variable results.

- Differences of opinions in how many vertebrae (levels) to fuse have potentially serious ramifications. One surgeon might want to fuse your spine down to L1, while another might go a level lower, to L2. Fusing just one more lumbar vertebra can have a significant, permanent impact on your bending flexibility and is a decision that should not be made lightly. In contrast, fusing an additional thoracic vertebra will probably not have a discernible impact on your flexibility but, even so, every additional vertebra that is fused extends your surgery a little longer, may mean a little bit more blood loss, slightly increases the risk of complications, and so on. There are always pros and cons to these kinds of decisions; you should discuss this in more detail with all the surgeons you are considering.

- Differences in what surgical approach to use (anterior, posterior, or both) are also important, but here the specific experience of the surgeon is critical. Your particular case may favor one approach over another, but if there is an option, you need to evaluate the surgeon's experience and track record of success in performing one approach over the other.

If the surgeons' opinions vary, you should take careful notes on the differences and then return to your preferred surgeon to discuss them. When you call to schedule this review, tell the receptionist that you may need more time than is usually allotted per appointment to review your case in sufficient detail. The two surgeons may discuss your case further to understand the differing opinions and reach consensus. Or, the two surgeons may simply agree to disagree. At that point, you have two options: you can either trust your instinct and choose the surgeon whose opinion makes more sense to you, or you can get additional opinions until you begin to feel that one approach is superior.

My experience may help illustrate the kinds of differences you may encounter. The first surgeon I saw, Surgeon A, had a solid track record and excellent credentials. He proposed performing a posterior-approach fusion of eight thoracic vertebrae down to one lumbar level. Surgeon B had less experience but otherwise excellent credentials. He concurred that a posterior approach would be most appropriate, but recommended fusing three levels higher and one lumbar level lower. He felt that not fusing higher would result in an imbalance in my shoulders, and not fusing lower would fail to correct my compensatory lumbar curve sufficiently. I went back to Surgeon A to discuss this. He concurred that my shoulders would initially be imbalanced, but in his experience this imbalance would correct itself over time. He also felt that the lumbar curve would correct enough on its own. The two surgeons ran into each other at a conference and discussed my case further. They acknowledged that neither of their two opinions was right or wrong— they were just different, and either surgeon would probably perform a successful surgery. My preference was to go with Surgeon A's more conservative approach and fuse as few vertebrae as possible. I was willing to take a small risk that additional surgery would need to be performed later in my life to extend the fusion higher or lower, in exchange for keeping more vertebrae free. As it turned out, I indeed had some imbalance in my shoulders, but over the span of a few months it disappeared, and my lumbar curve corrected 68% to a negligible 10° curve. I feel I made the right decision.

Choosing a Hospital

You need to ensure that all members of the surgical, preoperative, and post-operative staff that will be working with you have adequate training, experience, and the equipment necessary to treat scoliosis surgery patients. This combination is usually only found in larger hospitals in mid-sized to large cities. Of course, you may not have a choice of hospital. Your insurance may only cover surgeries performed at in-network hospitals, and there may only be one in your area that performs spinal fusions. Or, the surgeon you want to have perform your surgery may only be affiliated with one hospital. If you have a choice, it is definitely worth spending some time to investigate your options.

The best source of information is patients who have had spinal fusion surgery performed at a hospital you are considering. Ask them detailed questions about their experiences.

Another good place to start is with "hospital report cards." These are available online or in printed form from several sources and may reveal, for instance, that one hospital in your area performs far more spinal fusions than the other, or that the surgical complication rate for spinal fusions at one hospital in your region is lowest. *Health Grades* (www.healthgrades.com), for example, allows you to search for hospitals by geographic region and compare their performance on a variety of metrics for a specific procedure, including spinal fusions. *U.S. News & World Report* (www.usnews.com) has an updated list of the fifty best hospitals in the country for orthopedics, though this is not broken down by specific procedures. Also, your insurance provider may offer free access to databases that contain more comprehensive comparison information. This kind of information provides useful data but should not be the only factor in your decision where to have the surgery performed.

A visit to the hospital is a good idea. Inspect the facilities as much as you can. Most hospitals have a special floor or wing dedicated to orthopedic patients. Ask the nursing staff in that section to give you a tour of their facilities. This will give you an idea of the size of the rooms (where, after all, you will be staying for up to a week or more), how many nurses are on-call, and what other facilities are available. You may also be able to meet some of the hospital staff who would care for you while you are recovering. Remember that an important factor in determining where you will have surgery is the quality of the other medical professionals who will provide your care before, during, and after surgery. These include the anesthesiologist, radiologist, physical therapists, nurses, dieticians, and others. You should therefore take a holistic approach to finding the right combination of people to give you care.

You may be able to have specialists not affiliated with the hospital where you will have surgery provide you with care. For example, anesthesiologists can be independently affiliated. Surgeons usually have certain anesthesiologists they prefer to work with, but if you have a personal preference, the surgeon may be able to accommodate it. You might also opt to hire a private nurse or physical therapist instead of relying on the hospital's staff. Making substitutions such as these can drastically affect the quality of care you receive.

The hospital you prefer may be in a city far from your home. You should be willing to travel to receive the best surgery. However, traveling home from the hospital, whether by car or plane, can be an extremely painful experience. If the distance from your home to the hospital is particularly great, I would recommend you take this factor into account in selecting where you will have surgery. See *Traveling Home* in Chapter 6 for tips on making the journey tolerable.

Some hospitals will allow you to pre-register up to a week or so in advance of your surgery date. Pre-registration simply means providing basic information (address, emergency contact information, known drug allergies, etc.) and insurance coverage, and signing legal consent forms. You will also receive some important check-in procedures so you know where and when to appear on the day of surgery. If pre-registration is an option for you, I *strongly* recommend doing it. This will save you time on the day of surgery and, more importantly, removes one more thing to worry about on the day of surgery.

Setting a Date for Surgery

As discussed in Chapter 2, scoliosis surgery is almost never urgent. Unless you are in extreme pain or having serious breathing difficulties because of your curvature, you can usually safely delay surgery for months or even years. Remember, though, that there are some penalties for waiting too long. In general, the younger you are, the faster you will recover, the more correction can be achieved, and the lower the chance of surgical complications. On the other hand, surgical procedures may continue to improve as they have over the last twenty years. Waiting for one of these potential future procedures may get you improved correction, a faster recovery with less pain, fewer complications, or other benefits not yet known.

There are a lot of valid reasons to postpone having surgery. If you are female, you may wish to have a baby and raise it for a few years before surgery. If you are a student athlete, you may want to finish a sports season. If you are working, you may want to finish an important project or contract assignment. Maybe you need a couple of years to save enough money to afford the out-of-pocket costs of surgery. Perhaps you will be moving soon and want to have the surgery performed near your new home. Or maybe weddings, graduations, or other major events that are important for you to attend are forthcoming. In addition to these fairly obvious reasons to delay surgery, there are some less obvious issues to consider, which include:

Availability of caregivers. You will need day-to-day assistance once you are released from the hospital. Depending on how quickly you recover from surgery, assistance may be required for as little as two weeks or as long as six months. Your health insurance plan may cover home visits by nurses, but this is rarely sufficient. Ideally, you have a spouse, significant other, parent, or roommate who can help you. Perhaps you have family who live nearby or very generous neighbors. Whatever the case, you should attempt to schedule your surgery around *their* availability. You want to maximize the amount of time they can spend with you and, of course, be respectful of their schedules and priorities as much as possible.

Work and school. If you work or attend school, you should give careful consideration to the impact your post-surgical absence may have.

If you are employed, check to see whether your employer has a short-term disability plan in place. This can continue to give you a portion of your salary while you recover. If you have an office job, telecommuting may also be an option. Shortly after surgery, many patients will be able to process e-mail and have phone conversations from home, which may be sufficient for an employer to consider you still working full-time and thus continue to pay you at your normal wage. Travel, manual labor, and rigid hours will not be possible. If you are considering a career or employer change, this might be a good time to have surgery.

It is difficult to predict when one can return to school. Some young patients return to school just three weeks after surgery. Others may need to take off an entire semester. If possible, schedule your surgery for early in the summer, or right at the beginning of a long holiday (such as the Christmas/New Year break) to minimize the number of school days you will have to miss.

Your health insurance. If you don't have your own health insurance, perhaps the person whose insurance carrier covers you is considering a career change. If the next employer offers a better health plan, you may want to wait until that coverage becomes active to minimize your out-of-pocket expenses. Be certain, however, that your case of scoliosis will not be excluded as a pre-existing condition.

The weather. The majority of orthopedic surgeons will recommend you walk as much as possible after surgery. If you have a treadmill, walking indoors may be fine. If not, or if you prefer to walk outside, try to schedule surgery for a time of year when the weather is conducive to outside walking. If you live in a climate that is warm most of the year, this may not be a factor. For those who suffer from Seasonal Affective Disorder and need ample sunlight to avoid feeling depressed, winter can be a horrible time to have surgery.

Getting your life in order. As this and the next chapter illustrate, there are many things to do before undergoing surgery. You will probably need two months to do everything outlined here.

Scheduling Surgery Around Pregnancy

Scoliosis surgery in no way interferes medically with a woman's ability to conceive, carry, or deliver a baby. However, a woman who wants to have children needs to give additional thought about scheduling her surgery. The ideal time to become pregnant would be at least one year after surgery. Several things need to be considered:

- You cannot be pregnant at the time of surgery. There are too many potential complications for you and the risk to your child is not warranted.

- You do not want to become pregnant until after your spine is at least *mostly* healed—about six months after surgery. The added weight of an unborn child will place potentially harmful stress on your fragile spine.

- There are some reports of scoliosis progressing during pregnancy, but this has proved insignificant statistically. However, one study found that, compared to other patients, the curves of patients who had multiple pregnancies before age twenty were more likely to progress after bracing.

- You will need several x-rays taken of your back during follow-up visits with your surgeon during the first year after your surgery. There is some risk of damage to a developing fetus from x-ray exposure.

- The success or failure of your scoliosis surgery will usually become evident during the first year following your surgery. In the unlikely event that revision surgery is necessary or complications develop during this time, it would understandably be better not to be pregnant.

- If you have a lumbar fusion down to L5 or to the sacrum, an anesthesiologist may not be able to give you an epidural during childbirth. The epidural catheter must be inserted directly into the spinal column around L5, which may be blocked by the fused vertebrae.

- Very young children obviously require tremendous amounts of time and energy that you will not have while recovering from surgery. Holding young children in your arms can painfully strain your back while you are recuperating.

Paying For Surgery

Scoliosis surgery is extremely expensive. Total costs typically range from about $75,000 to $300,000. Unless you are unusually wealthy, you will need to pay for it by alternate means. Health insurance is obviously the preferred means of subsidizing the cost.

You will almost certainly need a pre-authorization from your insurance carrier before your surgery can be scheduled. Your surgeon's staff can arrange this. The pre-authorization process can go quickly or can take weeks, depending on the efficiency of your insurance carrier and to what extent the specifics of your surgical procedure may be considered unusual, unnecessary, or extreme. Insurance companies may deny coverage of specific aspects of your surgery. For example, some insurance companies will not cover experimental bone grafting techniques like BMP, or the use of titanium instrumentation (which is more expensive than stainless steel), even if your surgeon feels it is the best course of care in your case.

Insurance companies may also deny coverage for the expenses of certain surgical team members, such as those for a "surgical assistant," even though surgical assistants are routinely utilized. Your surgeon's staff is probably accustomed to debating with insurance carriers the merits of specific surgical procedures and the use of certain materials and staff members. Insurance carriers may change their initial position after discussing your case with medical professionals. Be aware that resolving the myriad complexity of claims, co-pays, deductibles, caps, and so forth can take months.

Insurance generally covers only some fixed percentage of expenses, so you will probably need to subsidize the difference with your own money or by taking out a loan. You need to be careful in estimating your total out-of-pocket charges when working with insurance carriers. The computation of benefits for inpatient surgery is seldom simple. For example, my PPO plan covered 100% of my surgical and hospitalization costs after I paid a $500 deductible and a $250 "per hospital confinement" charge. But in the end I paid more than $750 because other medical professionals who provided services associated with my surgery generated additional charges. For example, the anesthesiologist my surgeon preferred to work with was not affiliated with the hospital where my surgery was performed, so his services were not included in the $750 blanket charge. However, because the anesthesiologist was a member of my PPO network, my insurance carrier covered 90% of his charges. In contrast, my pathologist—the specialist responsible for all testing performed on me before and after surgery—was not part of my PPO network, so only 60% of his services were covered by my insurance.

You may be able to appeal this with your insurance company if something like this happens to you. In some cases, if you were an inpatient when medical services were rendered and you had no choice over who provided the services in question, insurance companies will not hold you accountable for those charges.

If you do not have insurance, or if your current insurance will not cover enough of your expenses to make the surgery affordable, you *may* be able switch to another insurance provider with better coverage. Better coverage plans will almost certainly have higher premiums (the amount you must pay each month to maintain coverage), but they may more than make up for this increase by providing you with substantial savings off the price of surgery. Note, though, that virtually every insurance plan other than the group plans offered by many employers will deny you coverage for pre-existing conditions. The definition of a pre-existing condition varies slightly from provider to provider, but generally it is any condition for which you sought treatment in the last one or two calendar years. In terms of scoliosis, that means that if you saw an orthopedist, orthotist, radiologist, or any other medical professional for your scoliosis in the last twelve months, you are ineligible for coverage. Some insurance plans will cover a pre-existing condition if you have been a member of that insurance provider for at least one year. Since scoliosis surgery is almost never urgent, this means that you may be able to switch to an insurance provider that will cover pre-existing conditions after one year, as long as you can delay your surgery for at least one year. *Before you do this, make absolutely certain that the provider will allow this.*

You have other options if you do not have insurance or other means to pay for surgery:

- Surgeons affiliated with scoliosis centers at some major teaching hospitals may perform the surgery at no cost to you or at a reduced rate, based on your financial need or your willingness to participate in a surgical research study.

- Medicaid will pay for surgery, if you are eligible. Eligibility requirements for Medicaid benefits vary by state. Contact the Centers for Medicare & Medicaid Services, 7500 Security Boulevard, Baltimore, MD 21244-1850, (410) 786-3000, or on the Internet at cms.hhs.gov.

- Shriners Hospitals in the following cities will perform scoliosis surgery on children up to eighteen years of age at no charge whatsoever: Chicago, Greenville (SC), Honolulu, Houston, Lexington (KY), Los Angeles,

Minneapolis, Philadelphia, Portland, Shreveport (LA), Spokane, Spring-field (MA), St. Louis, Tampa, and outside the United States in Montreal and Mexico City. Call (800) 237-5055.

- Texas residents under the age of 18 may be eligible to receive no-cost surgery at the Texas Scottish Rite Hospital for Children in Dallas. See www.tsrh.com or call (214) 559-5000 for more information.

- Banks may loan you the money to pay for surgery. Another option is to refinance your home with a "cash-out" mortgage.

- You may be able to borrow money from your retirement accounts, such as 401(k) or IRA plans. These plans usually allow you to withdraw funds without penalty if the money is to be used for medical costs not covered by insurance and exceed 7.5% of your adjusted gross income. You can also usually avoid a penalty if you are totally disabled.

Other tips to manage surgery-related expenses:

- Some hospitals offer payment plans that may ease your financial burden by spreading out payments over several months. Most hospitals will also allow you to place all charges on your credit card.

- All medical expenses related to your scoliosis treatment that are not covered by insurance are tax deductible, as long as these expenses exceed 7.5% of your adjusted gross income and you itemize deductions in lieu of taking a standard deduction (per 2004 tax law, which may change).

- You will receive one or more prescriptions for pain medication when you are discharged from the hospital. Almost all of these medications have a generic equivalent (a non-name brand). Ask your surgeon to allow generic substitutions, since most insurance carriers will charge you less for generic drugs. Your insurance carrier may also provide a discount if you order a 90-day supply of medications through a mail order house, but, depending on the medication, you may not be able to obtain large quantities of narcotic medication legally though the mail at one time.

Establishing a Support System

Undergoing and recovering from scoliosis surgery may be the hardest thing you will ever do. It is very difficult—some would argue impossible—to go through it on your own. It is therefore important that you establish a support system *before* having surgery to help you through the ordeal. You will need two kinds of assistance: emotional and physical.

Regardless of how strong-willed you are, you will need people to console you emotionally. Scoliosis surgery will stretch you to the extremes of your emotional and mental limits. In addition, once you are home recuperating, you will find plenty of things that need to be done that require physical strength that you will not have at first. Previously simple chores and errands, like taking out the garbage or buying groceries, will suddenly be difficult or impossible until you regain your normal strength. These two kinds of assistance may not be provided by the same people. You need to give some thought to who these people will be. You will find out who your true friends are.

Your supporters may be obvious—if you are married, or live with your parents, for example. But if you live alone or with someone who has significant time commitments, you may need to expand your search to include friends, neighbors, and colleagues.

Identifying people to help you with physical tasks is, for obvious reasons, a lot easier than building an emotional support base. Even if you have close friends who can provide you with ample emotional support, you may also find that it is useful to have some people in the group that have been through the surgery and know exactly what you are going through—even if these people are complete strangers. This is where online or in-person scoliosis support groups can be of great help.

A few thoughts and suggestions:

- *People are often more willing to help than you expect.* It is in some ways an honor to be asked for help by someone in need.

- *The more others know about your condition, the more they can help you.* Sharing this book with others is a good way to familiarize them with what you will be going through.

- *Understand others' schedules and constraints.* Do not expect anyone to be at your service anytime, day or night. Be realistic. Everyone has other commitments that they will try to balance with yours.

- *Be specific about how others can best help you.* Make sure others understand what they are getting into. Some people are admittedly better at, or more willing to, run errands for you than doing your laundry.

- *Forewarn others about your potential emotional state.* It would be courteous to let people know ahead of time that you may, at times, be inadvertently irritable towards them due to the emotional roller coaster you will be on while recovering. Apologize in advance.

- *Share your good news.* Tell others how they are helping you recover. Keep them apprised once you are back on your feet as to how you are doing. They will appreciate the feedback.

CHAPTER FIVE

Preparing for Surgery

In this chapter, you will find information that will help you prepare yourself, both physically and emotionally, in the weeks leading up to surgery. The suggestions below will help maximize your chances of a successful surgical outcome and a smooth recovery.

Preparing Yourself Mentally and Emotionally

Scoliosis surgery is, without a doubt, scary. In the days, weeks, and months preceding your surgery, you will probably struggle to confront the inevitable. This is especially true if you have never had any kind of surgery before or have never been hospitalized, and therefore do not know what to expect. How every person deals with fear, stress, and anxiety is unique. Here are a few suggestions that may prove valuable:

- Practice whatever relaxation techniques you know work for you. If you don't have a preferred means of controlling anxiety, you might want to go to a book store or library and browse through books on relaxation techniques or stress management or, alternatively, enroll in a short course on relaxation training.

- Talking to a professional therapist is a good idea if your anxiety interferes with your daily life

- Regardless of whatever else you do, exercise is a great daily habit to practice, as it both relieves stress and helps prepare your body physically for your postoperative recovery

- Start using your support system. Talk to your supporters about your concerns.

Preoperative Exercise, Diet, and Nutrition

Most orthopedic surgeons will not prescribe a specific exercise or nutritional regimen to patients about to undergo scoliosis surgery. Nonetheless, it is in your interest to get into the best physical shape you can prior to surgery. The stronger and healthier you are before your surgery, the faster and easier you will recover. Being in good physical condition can also alleviate stress and provide you with more mental stamina when confronting the prospect of surgery. You should consult your doctor before beginning any exercise, diet, or nutrition program.

Like any well-designed exercise program, you should combine aerobic conditioning with muscle conditioning. Do whatever aerobic activities you like—walking, bicycling, swimming, whatever—to get your heart and lungs in their best condition. For muscle conditioning, you should concentrate on building up strength in your upper arms and legs. This is because, while recovering from surgery, you will use the strength in your arms and legs to get in and out of bed and lower and raise yourself from chairs. You will also bend more from your legs than ever before, as your back will have impaired flexibility. You actually do *not* want to build up your back muscles, as these will be cut into during surgery.

If you are overweight, you should speak to your surgeon about whether losing weight prior to surgery should be a goal. Keep in mind that you may lose a lot of weight in the week or two following surgery, so having some extra "padding" can be a good and safe thing.

There are no specific foods that will better prepare your body for surgery. Follow common-sense guidelines and eat a healthy, well-balanced diet. You may want to add a multi-vitamin to your diet for a few weeks before (and after) surgery. Virtually every vitamin contributes in some way to your body's ability to repair itself after surgery, so raising the levels of these vitamins before surgery can only be beneficial. Some surgeons will also ask that you take iron supplements to maintain high iron levels in your body.

You should cease taking herbal supplements for several weeks prior to surgery. Some herbs are known or believed to interfere with anesthesia, and some may increase bleeding during surgery.

If you smoke heavily, you should quit at least three months prior to surgery. Smoking can negatively affect the integrity of a spinal fusion.

Donating Blood

You will lose some blood during surgery. The amount of blood loss is usually negligible, and losing blood in the controlled environment of an operating room is rarely cause for concern. However, just in case, you should have some extra blood on hand should a transfusion become necessary. To prepare for this contingency, your surgeon may encourage you to donate your own blood (called *autologous donation*) in advance of your surgery. If necessary, this blood will be replaced intravenously to compensate for any blood lost during surgery. This is safer than receiving blood from an anonymous donor through a blood bank. Even though all donated blood is screened for infectious diseases like the AIDS virus (HIV) and hepatitis, there is always a small chance that something will avoid detection. There is also a small chance that the blood type of anonymous blood will be mismatched to your own. Why take that risk?

Not everyone can donate blood. Individuals who weigh less than 110 pounds, people with anemia, and people who are in otherwise frail health are usually excluded. In these cases, you will need a blood transfusion using blood from a blood bank.

Blood removed from your body can be safely stored for up to six weeks prior to your surgery, or frozen for even longer periods of time. I would advise against waiting too long to donate blood, because if you become sick unexpectedly within three days prior to donating, you cannot donate. You do not want to put "sick blood" back in your body, especially after surgery when your body's resistance to any illness will be weak. By scheduling your donation roughly three weeks prior to your surgery date, you will have a comfortable margin of safety should you need to postpone your donation due to unexpected illness. Also note that you cannot donate blood during the week prior to surgery.

For the ten days prior to donating your blood, you should take over-the-counter iron supplements to raise your red blood cell count. Iron comes in many forms; *ferrous sulfate* is usually recommended, but ask your surgeon what type and dosage he or she recommends. Iron tends to be better absorbed if taken one hour before or within two hours after eating a meal. The addition of vitamin C may also improve iron absorption. Note that iron supplements can darken urine and stools, and may cause constipation. You should eat a good meal a few hours prior to donating blood, and drink plenty of water or other non-caffeinated beverages that day.

Note that certain medications cannot be taken within days or sometimes weeks prior to donating blood. Be sure to tell your doctor about all prescription and non-prescription drugs you are taking.

Donating blood is a straightforward process. Your surgeon will instruct you to make an appointment at a local facility such as a blood donation center or American Red Cross office that specializes in blood collection. At the center, you will fill out some paperwork, be interviewed to make sure you are relatively healthy, and your iron level will be tested via a quick finger pinprick test. A nurse or technician will then hook you up to a machine that will automatically withdraw blood from your arm. The entire process is virtually painless, though some individuals experience mild discomfort where the needle was inserted into the arm, or other symptoms like upset stomach, dizziness, and subsequent bruising where the needle was inserted. Some people faint, but this is rare. After your blood is extracted, you will be asked to rest at the facility for fifteen minutes or so while consuming sugar-rich foods and drinks. This will quickly raise your blood sugar level to replenish the energy loss most people experience after donating blood.

In most cases, you will need to donate two to four units of blood (one unit equals one pint). Most standard posterior or anterior surgeries require two units to be on-hand during your surgery; longer procedures require three or four; and very complicated surgeries may require six or more units. Generally, only a small portion of the blood you donate will need to be used, if any. In the operating room, some of the blood you lose may be "recycled" with a machine called a *cell saver*. This machine collects some of the blood you lose, filters it, and then returns it to your body.

One unit of blood can be extracted in about twenty minutes. The paperwork, interview, iron testing, and resting period can add another forty-five minutes to your visit. If you need to donate more than two units, you should schedule a second appointment. Donating more than two units in one visit may lead to marked weakness, and the visit itself becomes quite long and tedious. Younger patients may only be able to donate one unit per visit safely.

There are alternatives to autologous transfusions. You may be given a hormone called EPO (erythropoietin) just prior to surgery. EPO can raise your hemoglobin count to the point where blood loss is not a problem. There are also medications that decrease intraoperative bleeding. These alternatives are risky and expensive. Unless you have a compelling reason not to donate your own blood, you should by all means do so. One exception to this, however, is that the parents of a young child about to undergo surgery may wish to donate his or her blood to the child to avoid putting the child through added anguish, though this is only viable if the blood types are compatible.

Medications

You should inform your surgeon of all medications you are taking, including over-the-counter drugs. Many hospitals will allow you to bring prescription medications you are taking with you to the hospital. Most drugs will not interfere with your surgery and will not need to be discontinued prior to surgery. There are some exceptions, however.

One class of medication that you should avoid taking two weeks prior to, and three months after surgery, are non-steroidal anti-inflammatory drugs (NSAIDs) and similar drugs called COX-2 inhibitors. These include over-the-counter painkillers like ibuprofen (Advil, Motrin), naproxen sodium (Aleve), ketoprofen (Actron®, Orudis KT®, Oruvail®), and generic aspirin, as well as prescription painkillers like indomethacin (Indocin®), etodolac (Lodine®), celecoxib (Celebrex®), nabumetone (Relafen®), diclofenac (Cataflam®, Voltaren®, Voltaren-XR®), and tramadol (Ultram®), and others.

There are two problems with NSAIDs and aspirin: they can lead to increased blood loss during surgery, and there is some research to suggest that they may inhibit the fusion process postoperatively. It may seem that discontinuing the use of NSAIDs a full two weeks before surgery is premature, but traces of these drugs remain in the body for quite some time and even these small amounts can cause complications.

If you are taking aspirin or an anticoagulant (blood-thinning drug) like warfarin (Coumadin®) for your heart, talk to your doctor about whether and when you should discontinue taking it.

Getting Your House and Life in Order

Scoliosis surgery is a major interruption to your life. You will be in the hospital for several days, and then you will spend a few weeks or months recovering at home. During this time, you will face all kinds of physical challenges. It is hard to imagine living without bending your back or raising your arms, while at the same time being in some degree of pain and probably on pain control medication that makes you tired and dizzy. While you cannot avoid this challenge, there are steps you can take before surgery that will make your recovery much easier. See Appendix A for more suggestions.

Move frequently-used items up higher. For example, move pots and pans stored in under-counter cupboards to above-counter cupboards, or just place them on your countertop.

Make frequently-used switches more accessible. For example, if the on/off switch of your bedside lamp is difficult to reach without bending or stretching, attach the lamp to an extension cord with a switch and position it closer to your bed.

Clear paths. You may need more room than usual to navigate inside your house, especially if you need someone to assist you in walking or if you will be using a walker or cane. Remove easily breakable items in case you need to lean on the wall or on a piece of furniture. Secure, remove, or replace slippery surfaces like throw rugs on which you might slip.

Pre-pay bills two or three months in advance. An alternative is to set up automatic withdrawal for recurring payments like your mortgage or car payments. Making financial decisions while under the influence of painkillers can be a costly mistake.

Get predictable appointments out of the way. For instance, take your pets to the veterinarian for a checkup. Also be sure to take care of any routine medical appointments for yourself, such as annual gynecological exams or teeth cleanings. In fact, some dentists and other medical professionals will not work on you for at least six months following a major surgery because of your heightened susceptibility to infection. Even just for a routine teeth cleaning—which can release quite a bit of bacteria into your body—a dentist may require you to take a short course of antibiotics before and after your visit to minimize the risk of infection.

Preparing Your Body

As your surgery date approaches, there are few simple things you can do to minimize problems during and after surgery.

- *If you have not already done so, quit smoking!*

- *Taper off your consumption of alcoholic beverages and do not use illegal drugs.* You need your body to be in peak mental and physical condition prior to surgery.

- *Take good care of the skin on your back.* The incision site needs to be clean and wound-free. Cutting into damaged skin can lead to a serious infection. If you have a sunburn, rash, or sores on your back, the surgery must be rescheduled. If you have acne on your back, you should see a dermatologist a few weeks prior to surgery to get it under control. Avoid activities like contact sports that can result in bruising, scraping, or cutting the skin on your back.

- *Get a haircut.* You will probably not be able to get a haircut for some time after surgery. More importantly, you will not be able to wash your hair thoroughly for at least a week after surgery, so shorter hair will be easier to keep relatively clean.

- *For women, remove leg hair by waxing or other means.* Shaving your legs may be difficult or impossible for some time after surgery.

Preadmission Examinations and Testing

You need to be generally healthy to undergo surgery safely. If you are sick, surgery may need to be postponed. Therefore, a week or two before surgery, many surgeons will ask that a pediatrician evaluate younger patients, a family doctor examine middle-aged patients, and that a specialist examine anyone with a current or recent health condition. Teenagers and younger adults who are obviously in good health are usually not asked to be "cleared" for surgery.

Even if you are cleared for surgery, every patient will need *pre-admission tests* (also called a *work-up*). These tests are usually scheduled a few days or a full week before your surgery, and are conducted at your surgeon's office or at the hospital where the surgery will be performed. The exam usually consists of some combination of:

- A pulmonary function test (PFT) to evaluate your lung function
- An electrocardiogram (EKG) to evaluate your heart
- Blood testing
- Urine testing
- An EEG (electroencephalogram) test to check the nerve impulses that travel through your spine. This is done by sending small electrical impulses through wires attached to pads connected to your head and legs. This does not hurt.

If you have not had x-rays of your back taken recently (usually within the previous three months), these will be done at this time. Sometimes a medical photographer will also take pictures of you and your back for before-and-after-surgery comparison.

You may be given a hospital bracelet at this time to wear when you check-in to the hospital. Be careful not to damage this band and do not lose it. It identifies you and also matches you to your blood type. If you lose it, any blood samples taken will need to be re-drawn.

Some surgeons or the hospital staff will use this time to explain the surgery and various hospital procedures to you in more depth. You should use this opportunity to ask any questions or voice any concerns that you may have. You should tell the doctors or nurses about any allergies you may have to medications, foods, tape, or latex (rubber products). Other topics that may be covered in this meeting include the following:

- How to use a small breathing device called an *incentive spirometer*, or just *inspirometer*. This device exercises your lungs after surgery by making you cough and breathe deeply. Coughing and deep breathing are extremely important to help clear your lungs and prevent pneumonia.

- How to roll over after surgery. This is called *logrolling*. After surgery, you will need to turn over in bed by rolling like a log, keeping your body straight and rigid and turning your entire body at the same time.

- How to exercise your legs and ankles to keep the blood moving in your legs while you are recuperating

- How the hospital will monitor and treat your postoperative pain

You may also meet your anesthesiologist at this time. Be sure to tell him or her about any negative experiences you have had previously with anesthesia, such as an allergic reaction to a particular medication or nausea.

Final Consultation with Your Surgeon

You will probably have a final meeting with your surgeon in the last four weeks prior to surgery to review precisely what he or she expects to do, to answer any remaining questions you have, and to receive any special instructions. If your surgeon does not require such a meeting, you should request one.

Make sure you know what the surgeon intends to do, keeping in mind that surgeons *do* change their minds about surgical specifics and may not have informed you of these. Some patients use this time to voice their preference for things such as titanium versus stainless steel rods. Other patients want to discuss additional opinions they have received.

You should make sure you understand what the surgeon's involvement with you and your family will be in the hospital. Good questions to ask your surgeon include the following:

1. How long will my surgery take?
2. Will I see you in the hospital before surgery? How soon after surgery?
3. Who will inform my family or friends waiting in the hospital of my condition, and when?
4. Will I be placed in the intensive care unit (ICU) after surgery?
5. Will I be on a respirator after surgery?
6. Will I have a chest tube? For how long?
7. Will I be getting prescription drugs that I normally take for other conditions during my hospitalization?

You should also inform the surgeon at this time about any health problems you have had recently and any new medications you are taking.

The Day Before Surgery

You cannot eat or drink anything within the eight hours prior to surgery. This usually means that, if your surgery check-in is scheduled for 8 a.m., you cannot consume anything after midnight the night before. You should take this restriction very seriously. If anything is in your stomach when you go under anesthesia, you may vomit, defecate, or wake up terribly sick hours later. Also, as your stomach will essentially shut down for a few days after surgery, anything you consume just before surgery will sit in your stomach for that time. Some hospitals will ask that you give yourself an enema the night before surgery.

Avoid consuming salty foods or alcohol on the day before surgery. These can cause you to wake up dehydrated and craving water, which you cannot drink.

Some hospitals will order that you scrub your planned incision site (your back and possibly your pelvis, if bone grafts are to be taken from your hip) with an iodine solution. Iodine is a strong anti-bacterial medication that will help prevent infection. If you are allergic to iodine, tell the doctor or nurse; alternates are available.

You should pack a bag to take with you to the hospital. You will need very little. Recommended items include:

- *A robe.* The hospital will provide one, but you probably own a nicer one. You might also want to bring some loose-fitting pajamas or a nightgown, and some slippers with a grippy sole.

- *Basic toiletries.* Again, the hospital will provide you with things like a toothbrush and toothpaste, but bring better-quality ones that you prefer. You might also want to bring a hair brush, and men might want to bring an electric shaver for facial hair; shaving with a regular razor will be very difficult.

- *Portable music system.* Some people just cannot live without music, and music can be relaxing. Unlike reading, which takes more mental focus than you will probably have while on painkillers, listening to music is an easy way to get your mind off pain. Whatever you bring to the hospital, make sure it has headphones. Also, keep in mind that few hospitals will provide you with a safe place to store valuables, so you should be careful. Don't forget to pack extra batteries.

- *Clothes to wear when discharged.* Bring a change of clothes that is easy to put on so you can walk out of the hospital looking sharp. Because some people temporarily "puff up" after surgery, be sure to bring oversized clothes or clothes that are adjustable (such as stretch pants). Do not bring clothes that require you to lift your arms to put on.

- *One or two long cotton t-shirts* if you will have a postoperative brace.

- *Anything else you like.* Bring a few things that comfort you, like pictures of loved ones or stuffed animals. This is especially important for younger patients.

The most important thing you should do the day before surgery is to relax. Take the day off, free yourself of any appointments or commitments, and do something fun. This will not be easy but is very important. You come out of surgery feeling the way you came in.

The Day of Surgery

You will have very little to do when you wake up on the morning of your surgery. A few things to remember:

- Do not eat or drink anything that morning, including water

- Do not chew gum or chewing tobacco, and do not smoke

- If you must take a medication orally and your doctor clears you to do so, take it with a very small sip of water

- If you wore contact lenses overnight, take them out. Wear glasses to the hospital if you need them. If you are only mildly nearsighted, pack your glasses in your suitcase or just leave them at home; you won't need to see anything clearly in the hospital.

- Take a good shower. You will not be able to shower for at least a few days.

- Brush your teeth but be sure not to swallow any toothpaste or water

- Avoid applying any cosmetics, perfumes or colognes, or any other skin or nail care products

- Remove any jewelry or piercings

- Try to have a bowel movement. You will not have another one for several days.

- Try to relax and maintain a positive mindset

CHAPTER SIX

The Hospital Experience
from Admission to Discharge

Your stay at the hospital can be divided into five phases:

1. Preoperative procedures
2. Surgery
3. Postoperative recovery room and intensive care
4. Transfer to your own room
5. Discharge

This section examines each of these phases in detail. Note that procedures will differ slightly between hospitals.

Preoperative Procedures

Most surgeries will last only a few hours, so typically a patient will check-in to the hospital on the same day as the surgery. If the surgery will be particularly long due to its complexity (like many combined anterior/posterior approach surgeries), the patient may be asked to check-in the night before so that the surgery can begin early the next morning. The general steps include the following:

Check-in. Even if you have pre-registered, you need to inform the reception staff that you have arrived at the hospital. If you were not given one previously, you will be given at least one plastic bracelet to wear during your entire stay in the hospital. The bracelet identifies you, your age, and other key information.

Change clothes. You will have to remove all your clothes and put on a gown. You will be given a bag in which to place your clothes; the nursing staff can hold on to this for you, but it is safer to give it to a friend or family member who is with you at check-in. You may also be given socks to keep your feet warm.

Testing. Your vital signs (blood pressure, pulse, and temperature) will be checked to make sure you are in good health. A blood sample will usually be drawn to verify your blood type, and women may be checked for pregnancy. You may be given an EKG. You may also be required to take a urine test.

The preoperative room. You will be placed on a bed with rollers (a gurney). A drug (often Versed) is usually administered at this time, through an IV (intravenous tube) or by injection, to help you relax. Your vital signs may be checked again. Medical specialists, such as an anesthesiologist, may talk to you about your experience with surgery, your overall health, and other medical matters. Various monitors may be connected. From here, patients will be rolled to the operating room. (Some hospitals ask patients to walk into the operating room instead of being rolled-in on a gurney).

Your surgeon or other members of the surgical team may come speak to you at any point during these steps. Your surgeon probably answered all the questions you have about your surgery in previous meetings. The brief visits by the surgeon or surgical staff are in many cases more to alleviate fears and to answer questions from any friends or family members who may be with you. This is especially common for younger patients. Your surgeon might not speak to you at all prior to surgery if he or she feels that you are mentally and emotionally prepared.

At several points during this process, you may be asked the same information over and over again. I was asked a dozen times what my name was and what surgery I was there for. This is not because the hospital staff has a short memory or fails to write anything down; they are trying to avoid severe errors, and be glad they are! You have probably heard of nightmarish events in which people had the wrong surgeries due to confusion about identities and other basic information. The best way to guard against this is to check and re-check information.

The Operating Room

In most hospitals, intravenous drugs to help the patient relax before surgery are administered in a preoperative staging area. These medications can be so relaxing that the patient falls asleep before being wheeled into the operating room (the "OR"). This happened to me, actually. The last thing I remember was being wheeled down a hallway that connected the preoperative room to the OR. I remember watching the fluorescent lights on the ceiling whiz by as I lay on my gurney. The next thing I knew, I was awake and not sure if the surgery had started. For some, this can be a good thing. The operating room can be a scary place and can raise your anxiety level, which is the last thing you need. For others, it is comforting to see the operating room and the surgical team.

If you are still alert when you arrive in the OR, be prepared to find it noisy, bright, and cold. The surgical team will be busy preparing and talking to each other; they are not deliberately ignoring you, they are just focusing on their tasks at hand. The team usually includes one or two anesthesiologists, several nurses, the surgeon, and often an assistant to the surgeon. The anesthesiologist will talk you through the process by which you will be put to sleep. He or she will usually ask you to count down from ten. Most people do not make it past eight or seven. You will not remember the surgery, you will have no concept of the passage of time, and you will not dream.

While you are in surgery, a nurse or surgical assistant will typically notify any friends or family members waiting in a designated area of your condition at periodic intervals or whenever some surgical milestone is reached. Sometimes this is done in person, while in other cases this is done by telephone. A phone in the waiting room will ring and the caller will ask to speak to someone from your party. If the phone rings and a hospital employee does not answer it, by all means someone in your party should! Your friends or family should not expect an update for at least the first two hours after you enter the OR.

Postoperative Recovery Room

You will wake up in a room that has different names, depending on the hospital. Common names are post-op, PACU (post anesthesia care unit), the recovery room, or just "recovery." You will stay in this room typically for one to four hours and you will be closely monitored to ensure that you wake up without complications. Most hospitals will not allow your family or friends to see you during this time; if they do, it will only be briefly.

Post-op is for many patients and their families the scariest time of the entire surgical process. The good news is that you probably will not remember much of this experience. The bad news is that you will probably wake up groggy, disoriented, and nauseated. Some patients vomit. You will probably feel some pain or numbness, despite the heavy painkillers you will be on at this time. Your back will be so stiff that you will feel paralyzed—despite what it feels like, you are most likely <u>not</u> actually paralyzed. When you get your bearings, you will probably find that you are connected to several tubes and machines:

One or more IVs. You may have needles in either or both of your wrists and/or in your neck. Through these IV tubes you will be receiving painkillers (usually morphine or a morphine derivative), antibiotics, anti-nausea medications, saline solution, or other medicines and fluids. When your digestive system is able to tolerate food, these IVs will be removed and you will take medications orally.

Foley catheter. This is a tube placed deep into your urethra, the tube in your body through which you urinate. Most patients do not feel the catheter inside them, but moving the catheter around may cause some discomfort. This tube drains into a bag that will be hanging off the side of your gurney. You will have no sensation of urinating. Urine will simply drain out through this tube. The catheter will be removed when you are able to walk to the bathroom or have the coordination to urinate into a bedpan or other receptacle. Be sure not to pull on the catheter, kink the tube, or move the urine bag—all of these can injure you or cause other problems.

Oxygen mask. Many patients will have some trouble breathing immediately following surgery. To help you breathe, an oxygen mask will be placed over your mouth and nose, or nasal prongs will be placed in your nostrils.

Hemovac®. This is a tube that drains excess accumulated blood and other fluids from your spine to prevent blood clots. You will not feel this because it is connected to your back in an area that will be numb and probably flooded with painkilling medication.

Cardiac monitor. Small electrode pads placed on different parts of your body will be connected to computerized monitors that track your heart rate, heart rhythm, respiration, and oxygen saturation. A video display next to your bed will display this information.

Pressure stockings and pneumatic compression boots. Because you will remain relatively motionless for some time after surgery, there is a risk that blood clots will form in the veins of your legs due to inactivity. To combat this, nurses will encourage you to wiggle your toes and stretch your feet as much as possible. As an added precaution, you will have compression boots on your legs. These plastic boots are applied over tight, elastic pressure stockings. The boots are attached to a pump which repeatedly applies gentle pressure to your legs then releases it. This simulates muscle contractions in your leg as if you were exercising them, thereby increasing blood flow throughout your legs and preventing a clot from forming. The boots are a bit uncomfortable and the waves of pressure on your legs can be a bit annoying, but again, you will be so out of it that it really will not bother you much. The boots will be removed when you can walk.

Chest tube. If you had an anterior-approach surgery, a tube may be left in your chest to remove air, blood, or fluid from the area around your lungs. This will make it easier for the lungs to refill with air when you inhale.

Despite your disorientation, you may become aware of some strange yet common sensations:

Your throat may hurt, and your voice may be scratchy. This is a normal aftereffect of having an *endotracheal tube* (ET) placed down your throat during surgery. If you have ever watched the television show "E.R." and seen a patient "intubated," you know what this looks like. The ET is connected to a respirator controlled by the anesthesiologist. He or she can accurately control your breathing using this system. This tube is usually removed before you wake up, but in some cases—particularly for very long surgeries—the tube will be left in your throat until the anesthesiologist verifies that you have woken up safely. Any throat irritation you experience is temporary and will dissipate on its own. Nurses may give you ice chips to help soothe your throat.

You may have "pinpoint" pain in areas of your body other than your back. This is a common effect of having been laying motionless face-down (posterior surgeries) or on your side (anterior surgeries) on an operating table for hours. These tables support your body at specific points on your arms and legs. The extreme proportion of your weight placed on these small number of points can cause pain that resembles the feeling of a bruise. The pains will go away on their own eventually, but it can take weeks.

You may be swollen in various parts of your body. Your entire face, eyes, lips, or other parts of your body may be swollen. This is normal and temporary. You may want to warn any family members or friends who are coming to visit you in the hospital about this, as it can be frightening for them.

Your back may itch. The surgeon will have probably covered your incision using dozens of Steri-Strips®, which are like small band-aids. These can itch or cause a rash. You may actually be allergic to the adhesive on the strips, in which case you may need to take antihistamines or apply a topical cortisone cream; discuss this with your surgeon. The incision itself can itch, too. It is very important that you do not scratch at your incision or peel-off the Steri-Strips before your incision has healed.

Intensive Care Unit

Once you are cleared by an anesthesiologist to leave the post-op room, you may be transferred to an intensive care unit (ICU) if your surgery necessitated a chest tube, if you have some complications worth monitoring, or if you reacted badly to the anesthesia. Not all hospitals separate the post-op room from ICU; these may be the same room. As a matter of policy, some hospitals route every postoperative patient to the ICU for a mandatory monitoring period. Stays in the ICU can be as short as twenty-four hours or as long as four or more days. As in the recovery room, your memories of the ICU will be hazy and you will most likely sleep through most of it.

In the ICU you may first feel significant pain, or at least significant discomfort. The pain will probably not be as severe in your spine as in the surrounding areas of your back. If you had a posterior-approach surgery, your surgeon may have injected a morphine derivative called Duramorph® directly into your spinal column. This will numb your spine significantly for up to twenty-four hours after surgery, but use of Duramorph has some risks. The drug may cause breathing problems and urinary retention, and it may mask neurological complications resulting from surgery. These are the kinds of things the ICU staff will be monitoring closely. When the Duramorph wears off, you will become more acutely aware of pain in your spine.

If you are reasonably coherent in the ICU, you may be introduced to a few techniques that you will need to utilize for the remainder of your hospital stay. These include:

Logrolling. It is important to keep your body moving to prevent blood clots and bedsores. Unfortunately, you will feel so stiff and sore that you will be unable to move your back. Therefore, nurses will "logroll" you. Two nurses will gently lift one side of the bed sheet under you, causing you to slowly roll over on one side. The trick is to get your hips, back, and shoulders to all turn at the same time. Once you are on your side, they will place pillows behind or under you to prop you up. They may do this back-and-forth to give you a full range of motion. It hurts, but you will get used to it quickly. Another reason to logroll you is to allow nurses to check your incision site and dressings for bleeding or other problems. They may need to do this at fixed time intervals, usually every two to four hours.

Breathing exercises. Your lungs will probably be weak after surgery due to the anesthesia and, if you had an anterior-approach surgery, due to the intentional deflation of one lung. Virtually all patients who have just had surgery will experience some temporary difficulty breathing. Breaths will feel shorter and more shallow than normal.

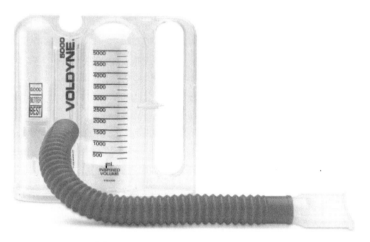

Figure 18: A typical inspirometer
Courtesy of Hudson RCI

To rebuild the strength in your lungs, prevent them from collapsing, and to prevent pneumonia, you will be asked to "exercise" your lungs using a plastic device called an *incentive spirometer*. This is also called an *inspirometer*, *volumetric exerciser*, *incentive breathing exerciser*, or *IBE*. All you need to do is take a deep breath, hold it as long as possible, and then exhale into the mouthpiece at the end of the tube as hard as you can. The tube is connected to a meter which will display the volume of air you are moving. There is no specific minimum number of times you should repeat this exercise, but it is in your interest to do it as much as you can tolerate. You do not need to have a nurse present, though sometimes a nurse will ask you to use the inspirometer in front of him or her to check how much air you are moving.

Coughing. Mucus collects in your lungs while laying down. This is not normally a problem, but in some cases this build-up can lead to pneumonia. The mucus build-up will also contribute to your breathing difficulties and the inspirometer exercises will help alleviate this. You should try to cough once every hour or so to clear out any mucus. It will hurt to cough, but it is a good, simple precaution to take.

Wiggling. As you will quickly learn while recuperating from scoliosis surgery, any and all motion will be helpful, even if it hurts. Moving is the first step on your path to recovery. This will help prevent bedsores and blood clots. While you will not initially be able to move your back, you will still have limited mobility in your legs and arms which will increase quickly with time. Use this to your advantage. Whenever possible, wiggle your toes, stretch your hands and feet, gently turn your legs—do *whatever* you can that does not hurt too much.

Visitors are almost always allowed in the ICU. Friends and family may have seen you briefly after surgery, but the first time they will really get to talk to or spend time with you will be in the ICU. They should be prepared to be a little unnerved. My mother recalls that the first time she saw me after surgery, my eyes were swollen and tearing, I could barely breathe, the Hemovac was filling with blood, I had IVs in his neck and arms, and my paleness was extreme. I was hooked up to monitors in the recovery room, where my mother saw that my blood pressure was too high, my pulse too fast, and my lung capacity too low. I was wheezing and breathing through an oxygen mask. Of course, I was not aware of any of this, and I quickly improved.

You will be extremely groggy and perhaps even delirious for up to forty-eight hours after surgery. You will probably not be able to hold a coherent conversation with anyone and you might say some awfully strange things, too. Although I have no recollection of this, I was apparently quite upset that a mariachi band had not yet arrived at the hospital. I also claimed to a doctor that I had hatched from an egg. At one point, I was convinced that I was in a business meeting that had gone terribly wrong. If there is a comical side to scoliosis surgery, this is it.

Your Hospital Room

You will be moved to your own hospital room twenty-four to forty-eight hours after surgery, barring any extreme surgical complications. You will be glad to be moved to your own room. Recovery rooms and ICUs are loud, confusing places. Having a little more quiet and privacy will feel great, especially because the time when most patients are moved to their own room is about the time they begin to "get with it."

The Day-to-Day

Most patients will remain in their assigned hospital room for three to five days. There will be a routine you will follow. Nurses and other hospital staff members will frequently enter your room, for a variety of reasons:

- To check your blood pressure, temperature, and pulse at fixed intervals every few hours. The oxygen level in your blood will be checked using a *pulse oximeter*, a small clip that attaches to your finger.
- To draw blood samples once or more per day
- To check your hands, legs, and feet for strength, numbness, tingling, or any other problem that could indicate a neurological complication from surgery
- To check your incision site once or more per day for signs of bleeding or infection, and to change dressings (bandages and Steri-Strips) if dirty
- To ask you to rate your pain level on a scale of one to ten. If necessary, they will advise your surgeon and may adjust the type and dosage of painkiller in your PCA (see *Pain Control*).
- To periodically check your respiratory performance using the inspirometer
- To empty the bags into which your catheter and Hemovac drain
- To change your bed sheets
- To do some personal grooming for you
- To clean your room

If necessary, nurses will wake you to do all of these things. This makes getting a solid block of sleep impossible, but you may have so much trouble sleeping anyway that you will not object.

You will have a call button by your bed with which you can summon a nurse if you need anything. I recommend you find out when the nursing shift changes and try to avoid asking for anything that is not urgent when a new shift starts. You will typically get a faster response once the new shift has settled into its routine.

Eating

Your body will temporarily shut down your digestive processes after surgery. As a result, you will initially be unable to digest solid food, so at first you will be given only liquids, then soft foods (such as Jell-O®, pudding, ice cream, and applesauce), then move up to regular food as your stomach starts functioning again. If you eat before your intestines are working, you may become bloated, nauseated, or vomit. You will be able to tell when your intestines start "waking up." You will hear churning sounds, feel stomach pangs, or pass gas. Hunger is a good sign, too.

Once you are able to eat solid foods, you will be served three meals a day at approximately the same time every day. Most patients will have little appetite and may feel perpetually nauseated, but it is important that you eat as much as you can to give your body the nutrients it needs to heal.

If you are not eating enough, an on-staff dietician may come talk to you. The dietician can order the hospital kitchen to serve you specific foods that you prefer, or have them prepared a certain way.

Pain Control

You will be in pain while recuperating in your hospital room. The pain may be intermittent, mild or severe, and may be more like soreness and discomfort than what you think of as pain—but the point is, you will definitely experience *some* degree of pain. Most people will have pain in a few places: the incision site (back and/or front and sides), the grafting site (ribs or pelvis, unless you did not have allograft bone taken from your body), and sometimes your stomach (due to the temporary shutdown of your digestive system). The muscles throughout your back will almost certainly hurt, too, as they adjust to their new configuration.

To control your pain, you will probably be connected via an IV tube in your wrist or arm to a computerized machine called a PCA (patient-controlled analgesia). The PCA automatically dispenses the pain medication specified by your surgeon. The PCA is usually programmed to deliver a continuous low-dose flow of pain medication. This flow of medication is usually enough to suppress most of the pain you will experience. If you are still in pain, however, or if you are about to engage in some activity that may temporarily increase your pain (such as walking), you can press a button on a hand-held control that will instruct the PCA to deliver a supplemental dose of medication. You will hear a beep when the button is pressed properly. You will feel the effect of the medication within a few minutes. Your doctor limits the amount of medication that the PCA can deliver within any timeframe, so it is impossible to overmedicate yourself.

Although it is perfectly acceptable for another caregiver by your side to press the button for you, only you should determine whether the button should be pressed. Do not let someone else assess *your* pain. Also, do not let someone else press the button while you are sleeping. This can cause fatal respiratory depression.

When your stomach is able to tolerate food, your IV connection to the PCA will be removed, and you will switch to taking medications by mouth. The nursing staff will control the dispensing of these medications. Your doctor will determine the dosage and frequency at which you will be given oral medications. If all runs smoothly, a nurse will come to your room at fixed intervals to give you the medication. Of course, in the real world, nurses may run behind schedule or will simply fail to show up. If this happens, you should press the intercom button on your bed to alert a nurse that you need your medications. Be assertive about your need for pain control.

I strongly recommend you double-check every medication given to you. Politely ask the nurse giving you the medication (whether intravenously or in a pill form), "What drug is this, and what is it for?" This will help prevent you from receiving the wrong drug accidentally, and should also prevent you from taking drugs you do not need. At one point while I was recovering, a nurse gave me a pill without any explanation. "What's this?" I asked. "It's for nausea," she replied. I told her that I was not the slightest bit nauseated and did not want it. She was fine with that. The same is true for painkillers—if you are really not in pain, do not take painkillers unnecessarily.

Your First Steps

Physical therapy will usually begin on day 2 or 3, the second or third day after your surgery. Your first goal should be simply to sit upright in bed. Some therapists will suggest you go a little further and try to dangle your legs over the edge of the bed. Even doing just this much may make you feel dizzy or nauseated. If you feel ready, try to stand up, even if for a moment. You will probably need someone's help to stand and, once standing, you will probably need to lean against a walker because you will have some trouble balancing. A staff physical therapist will most likely be holding on to you. Your therapist might also suggest you try sitting in a chair in your room instead of getting back into bed. At this point in your recovery, it may be better to sit upright than lay down. You need to get used to gravity again. Take things slowly. There is no reason to hurry or to push yourself too hard.

If you feel ready to take a few steps, go for it. Few patients can walk more than a few minutes the first time they try this. You will probably still have an IV attached to you; the IV unit has wheels on its base, and the therapist will "drive" it for you. Walking will feel very strange. Your leg muscles will feel weak from lack of recent usage. The correction of your spine may have re-centered you, so your center of balance may seem a bit off even though it is most likely better than before. If you had a bone graft taken from your hip, you may have a limp due to pain in your hip. If you had vertebral discs removed as part of your surgery, you may lean forward slightly. You may also lean to one side. Of course, some patients need time to adjust to being straighter; many scoliosis patients have leaned to one side most of their lives and now suddenly do not. You may feel that you are taller. You probably are! Straightening a crooked spine can add as much as two inches of height to a typical patient. If you have been the same height for years, suddenly being taller makes walking a little challenging at first because your center of gravity is higher. And complicating all of this is that you will be on painkilling drugs that contribute to feelings of dizziness, and you will still be tired from the entire surgical ordeal. You will feel as if you are learning to walk all over again, but remember, all of these new physical sensations are normal and temporary.

In addition to the strange physical experience of walking, you may also experience some very mixed emotions. It may hit you hard that things that you once took for granted are all of a sudden major challenges. Something as seemingly simple as walking down a hallway can be a big experience. You will have to think deliberately about every step you take. You will be surprised how slowly you need to walk and how much assistance you need. Do not be discouraged by small setbacks. Again, these are only temporary. While it is normal to feel discouraged at this time, try to keep things in perspective: you just had major surgery, and you are walking. That is no small accomplishment!

On day 3 or 4, your physical therapist will probably encourage you to walk as far as you can. Most patients are surprised how much easier this is with just one more day of recuperation. You may be eager to try walking because you are tired of laying in bed and want to return to a "normal" life as quickly as possible.

The difference in how you feel in the next one or two days can be astonishing. Some patients make such a drastic improvement, literally overnight, that they are released on day 4 or 5. Adults, or those who have had particularly long or complex surgeries, usually will need to stay in the hospital one to three more days. Even so, you will improve considerably during this time. By day 5, most if not all of your IVs and your catheter will have been removed. The lingering effects of your anesthesia will have subsided, so you will have more energy and will be more alert.

Walk as much and as often as you can during this time. Sit up in bed, or move to a chair. It may hurt to move, but the more you move, the less it will hurt. This is a paradox that you must embrace.

Visitors in the Hospital

You may want all your friends and family to come visit you in the hospital, but you need to give this some careful thought before you have surgery. There are some important reasons to limit visitations. First, visits can be disruptive while you are recuperating. You will want to sleep most of the time and visitors—or even the anticipation of a visit—can keep you awake. I fell asleep on some of those who visited me and felt guilty that they came all the way to the hospital to see me and yet we did not exchange more than a few passing words.

Another reason to minimize visitors is that you cannot always control what you say while you are groggy and under the influence of narcotics. This can hurt feelings and strain relationships. At one point in the hospital, I quite brashly told my girlfriend to go away. This understandably upset her and I do not even remember the incident.

A third reason to avoid too many visitors is that some people will frankly be shocked or even scared to see your physical condition. Postoperative recovery is not a good place for the squeamish or for children. There may be bags of your blood and your urine hanging from your hospital bed, you may be swollen in various places on your body, you may be pale as a ghost, you may need to vomit occasionally, and so on.

Also note that some hospitals do not allow visitors under a certain age because of the higher-than-normal rate of infections or viruses they may carry.

Of course, some visitors can certainly cheer you up. I can offer three recommendations:

- Do not allow any visitors other than close friends or immediate family members to visit you for at least three days after surgery, or at least one day after you get your own room, whichever occurs first. Before this time, you will be a mess physically and mentally and any visitations will not be useful to you nor enjoyable for your visitor.

- Schedule a set time for visitations. Do not tell your friends to "show up anytime." I recommend late afternoon visits because you will be at your worst early in the morning and will typically have the bulk of your tests, housekeeping, and exercise up until the mid-afternoon. If you will have a physical or occupational therapist working with you, make sure to find out what times he or she is available and be sure to schedule visitations around this.

- Tell your visitors what to expect ahead of time. This way, they will at least be partially prepared for your physical and mental state.

Postoperative Bracing

A small percentage of surgical patients will need to wear a brace around their torso for three to twelve months after surgery. The purpose of the brace is to provide additional support to patients whose backs will be particularly frail after surgery. This is typically indicated for older patients whose bones are weaker, or for those who have had particularly complex revision surgeries. Some surgeons, however, recommend that all of their postoperative patients wear a brace.

The most common type of brace for those who have had scoliosis surgery is called a TLSO, which stands for *thoracic lumbar sacral orthoses*. These are made of lightweight fiberglass and are either custom-made from a plaster mold of your body or, alternatively, an off-the-shelf brace may be used. Because your body dimensions will change as a result of the surgery, a custom-made brace must be fitted *after* your surgery, often while you are still in the hospital. This is usually done a few days after your surgery or whenever you are able to lie on a special molding table which takes an imprint of your body dimensions. It will then take another few days before the brace is made. Those who need a brace must therefore stay in the hospital a few days longer while the brace is made.

Some patients need to wear the brace full-time, while for others it is only necessary to wear the brace while doing upright activities to help counter the effect of gravity. You do not need to sleep or bathe in it. You will need to wear long t-shirts under your brace to absorb perspiration; you should buy several before entering the hospital. Most patients will find the brace uncomfortable or constricting at first, but many patients appreciate the extra support for their sore backs. The brace will do some of the work that your back muscles normally do in helping to keep you upright. This is great when your back muscles are sore from surgery, but during the months that you will wear the brace, those muscles will begin to atrophy. As a result, when you cease wearing the brace, your back will usually ache for a while when those muscles need to do any heavy lifting on their own. Patients will thus need to exercise or get physical therapy to rebuild their atrophied muscles.

Discharge from the Hospital

Your surgeon will determine when you can go home based on several criteria. Generally, you can be released when your vital signs are normal, your intestines are functioning, you are able to walk, your pain is in control, and you have no surgery-related complications that need to be monitored further. If there is no medical reason to keep you in the hospital, you will do just as well recovering at home.

Before you leave, either a nurse, your surgeon, or someone on your surgeon's staff will review discharge instructions with you and sometimes your family or other caregivers if they are present. These will typically instruct you not to bend, twist, or lift anything more than a few pounds, not to take a bath for a few days, and other instructions. The next chapter reviews many of the most common details.

You will also be given one or more prescriptions for painkillers and sometimes muscle relaxants to alleviate back spasms that some patients experience after scoliosis surgery. Be sure to ask about known side effects of these medications or possible interactions with any other drugs you are taking. Some surgeons will instruct you to continue taking iron supplements if you have been taking them for some time due to anemia.

Your surgeon will need to sign a discharge order that authorizes the hospital to release you. Once signed, most hospitals will let you leave whenever you are ready. Hospitals are not like hotels; there is no "check out" time. Take your time getting dressed and collecting your belongings. You may take things that the hospital has given to you, such as the inspirometer (you paid for it, after all) and anything else you need; if you feel queasy, for example, take a basin and a towel with you in case you vomit on the ride home.

Virtually every hospital has a policy that it must take you from your room to the hospital exit by wheelchair, even if you are able to walk. Enjoy this smooth ride, because the journey home will not be so pleasant.

Getting Home

Traveling home from the hospital after surgery can be extremely painful, even for short distances. You will feel every bump during a car ride as a jolt to your fragile spine. Simply sitting upright for a while may make you profoundly fatigued, dizzy, or nauseated. Make no mistake: there is absolutely no way you can drive yourself. You will still be in some degree of pain, and you will probably be on medications that will impair your driving abilities. Simply moving your arms to steer would be painful.

If you intend to travel by car, I would recommend at least a mid-size car, with reclining seats. Even better would be an SUV or van that is easier to get into and out of than a car. A vehicle with a softer suspension would also be preferable to one with a stiffer ride. If the distance is particularly long, or if your surgery was particularly complex such that sitting in an upright position would be too painful, you might consider renting a recreational vehicle equipped with a bed on which you can lie.

If the distance to the hospital is so great that flying becomes your only option, I recommend you buy a seat in first or business class. Seats in these sections are more comfortable, wider, and recline further. These seats are expensive, but you may find sitting in the more cramped coach class to be unbearable. You may want to use any frequent flyer miles you have accumulated to purchase an upgrade. A less expensive alternative would be to sit in an exit row seat, where at least you will have more legroom. Explain your situation to the gate agent when checking-in. He or she will let you board before the masses so you will not feel rushed, and may even upgrade you to first or business class for no extra charge if space is available. In addition, if the flight has ample free seats, the gate agent may be able to give you your own row so you have more space to stretch out.

Whether traveling by vehicle or plane, you should have some pillows on hand to support your head or back. And be sure to wear your seat belt.

CHAPTER SEVEN

Recovery, Coping, and Getting On With Your Life

Recovering from scoliosis surgery is a long-term process with three basic phases:

1. Recovery from the initial trauma of surgery (three to seven days after surgery)
2. Initial adjustment period while recuperating at home (one to three weeks after surgery)
3. Rapid daily improvement (three weeks after surgery and onward)

Chapter 6 explored the first phase, the "hospital stay." This chapter examines the second and third phases—the slow, often painful, process of getting your life back to normal.

Keeping Perspective

The most important thing to understand about recovering from scoliosis surgery is that it is not a linear process. You may feel better one day, then worse the next. Or, one thing may improve while something else gets worse. These up-and-down swings are normal as your body struggles to heal itself. Rapid improvement often comes in phases, separated by plateau periods during which the rate of improvement will seem to taper off or simply stop.

It is normal to feel discouraged by this. You would, of course, prefer a steady progression of improvement in every respect. I can offer three suggestions on coping with this. First, focus on the big picture. Whether or not it is readily apparent, you are most likely getting a little better every day *overall*.

Recovery from scoliosis surgery can be like the old "two steps forward, one step back" saying. Going back a step is frustrating—but you are still one step ahead of where you last were.

Secondly, continuously remind yourself just how far you have come in a short time. Think about how you felt when you first awoke from the anesthesia, then compare that to how you feel at the present time. Be patient.

Finally, call on the support system you established prior to surgery. You will need these people the most once you are home recuperating. They can help you in a variety of ways. Activities that benefit both them and you are best. For example, they could bring a video to your house and watch it with you. Or they could take a walk with you, which gives them some exercise, as well. You may of course have more pressing needs for less enjoyable things, such as taking out garbage or doing laundry. But it is worthwhile for you to try to find a balance of activities that only benefit you and things that are mutually enjoyable for both of you.

You also need to be an active participant in your recovery. Your body will heal itself, but you need to push yourself to help it along. The trick is not to push too hard. You need to continue to reaffirm a paradox that you learned in the hospital: you will feel better faster by doing the things that hurt. The hardest thing to do will be the best thing for you: move. It is all too easy to stay in bed or watch television all day while recuperating. Nothing could be worse for you. Research shows—as do thousands of testimonials from people who have gone through scoliosis surgery—that movement helps your body heal. It also makes you feel much better, mentally as well as physically. It does not matter precisely what you do or how often, but your goal should be to *move as much as you comfortably and safely can.* Laying in bed is fine, but try to turn over or stretch as often as possible. Take breaks while watching television. Take a quick stroll around your house. Stretch your legs, wiggle your toes, do anything except remain motionless for long periods of time.

This may not sound so bad if you are reading this before you have surgery, but trust me, the temptation to remain dormant will be powerful. Impeding your desire to move will be extreme fatigue and a host of other physical problems. You can overcome some of these with a positive mental attitude. It also helps to ask others around you to motivate you, in the same way that going to the gym is easier when others are meeting you there. If possible, get your friends and family to be your coaches and personal trainers. Taking daily walks with your caregivers is a great way to do this; everyone needs exercise, it is relaxing, and it is a great time to talk to people who care about you and your emotions.

Defining "Recovery"

One of the most common questions patients ask their surgeons prior to scoliosis surgery is, "How long will it take for me to recover?" There is no short answer to this question, because everyone recovers at a different rate and your recovery will be in stages. It is rare that a person wakes up one day and proclaims himself or herself "recovered." It is more likely that your recovery will be like climbing stairs, with each stair representing some important milestone. How high that staircase is depends on your physical condition prior to surgery and the complexity of the surgery you have had. Your surgeon may try to predict how quickly you will reach certain milestones, but surgeons are seldom accurate in this respect.

To give you some *rough* ballparks, most patients universally agree that the first three weeks after surgery are hell. There seems to be something magical about the three week mark. Younger patients are sometimes able to return to school at this time. Older patients frequently report far fewer problems at this point, though most cannot return to work for at least another three weeks. This is not to say that one is fully recovered after three to six weeks. Virtually everyone will still have some issues, such as occasional pain, difficulty sleeping, or diminished energy levels relative to their abilities prior to surgery. I do think it is fair to say, however, that for the majority of cases, 80% of the recovery battle will be fought in the first six to eight weeks after surgery.

Another way to define "recovered" would be the point at which you can return to normal activities. This depends on what normal activities you engaged in prior to surgery. Athletic patients will find that recovery in this sense will take several months. Most sports, especially contact or high-impact sports and exercises, must be avoided for four to six months after surgery. Remember, it can take a year or more before your spine is solidly fused and able to absorb significant impact. In contrast, if you led a relatively sedentary lifestyle prior to surgery, you will obviously be able to return to this quickly after surgery.

Initial Restrictions

When you are discharged from the hospital, your surgeon or a physician assistant will give you a sheet of instructions to follow over the next few weeks as you recover at home. The instructions will be personalized to your specific situation, but several instructions are almost universally common to all people recovering from scoliosis surgery. These include the following:

Do not bend over or twist. In general, you want to minimize activities that require you to move your torso—leaning, reaching, or stretching. Excessive torso motion may cause pain or, in extreme circumstances, dislodge hardware from the healing vertebrae.

Do not lift anything more than ten pounds or so. Medical professionals may debate the exact maximum weight one can safely lift, but five to ten pounds is the typical range. For reference, a gallon of milk weighs 8.6 pounds. If you must lift something, face the object and use your arms and hips as much as possible—do not exert force on your back muscles.

Keep your incision site(s) clean. The Steri-Strips, if applied to your incision, will fall off within one to three weeks. Do not touch them. Your surgeon may specify that you do not take a bath or otherwise completely submerge your incision site in water for at least two weeks. Showering once you get home is usually fine, as long as you avoid drenching the incision area. Do not direct a forceful water stream at the Steri-Strips, as this may loosen their adhesive. Some orthopedists will advise you to wait ten days to three weeks before completely submerging yourself in a bath.

Restrict exercise to walking. It is imperative that you walk as much as you can. Start with short, slow walks. You may want to have someone accompany you in case you feel dizzy and need assistance. You may need a cane or walker to support you. Gradually increase your distance and pace. As for other activities, my surgeon said it well: "avoid activities in which you might crash." For the first few weeks, do not ride a bike, skateboard, roller blade, ice skate, ride horses, do any contact sports, skydive, ski, or engage in similar activities—you most likely will not have the strength, anyway. You also need to avoid activities that cause impact to the spine, such as running, and avoid any resistance exercises (weight lifting) that stress your back. Most people can resume all of these activities in four to six months. Use your common sense.

At follow-up visits with your surgeon over the first year or two after your surgery, he or she may lift restrictions on specific activities based on your recovery progress. When considering whether it is safe to pursue a particular activity, the most important thing is always to defer to your own judgment and common sense.

Common Problems

Everyone will recover at a different rate and will have their own unique experience. However, the combined experiences of many scoliosis surgery patients suggests that there are some experiences common to all:

Pain. It is interesting that some patients report little or no pain in the hospital. This may be due to the strength of intravenous morphine or to the generalized numbness most people feel after surgery. Once they get home, everyone experiences some pain, but everyone experiences it differently. For some, it is an intense, agonizing feeling, while others are not quite sure that "pain" is really the right word. Many people describe how they feel as sore, stiff, uncomfortable, or achy.

You may also feel pain in different parts of your body, in different ways. If you have had a bone graft taken from your pelvis, your hip may feel sore. If you have undergone thoracoplasty, it will feel like you have broken ribs (you do!). The incision on your back or side may tingle or burn, almost like a paper cut. Many patients do not actually feel pain in their spine, though they do feel tension, soreness, numbness, or other types of discomfort in the muscles surrounding it.

Fatigue, weakness, and dizziness. Your body will expend an unbelievable amount of energy repairing itself. This will leave you feeling tired and weak. Compounding that, you will have trouble sleeping, which will prevent you from getting sufficient rest to feel energized. To make matters worse, you will probably be taking narcotic painkillers, which have the common side effect of making you tired and sometimes dizzy. Furthermore, some of your muscles will have partially atrophied due to lack of use while you were in the hospital, so using them again can cause further fatigue in addition to soreness.

For the first few weeks after surgery, you will need to plan your daily activities around the possibility that you will run out of energy at any point. Assume that you will need brief periods of rest (laying down or in a reclined seating position) throughout the day. If you have to perform big tasks, spread them out across the day; clean one room per day, not the entire house. Avoid beginning activities that you cannot stop at any time.

Sleep problems. Many things will prevent you from sleeping well. Foremost, you will be constantly uncomfortable physically. This makes laying down and remaining relatively motionless for long periods of time virtually impossible. You will be able to cat-nap, but it takes most people a few weeks to reach the point where they can get a solid, restful eight hours of continuous sleep. Lack of sufficient deep sleep may cause you to have some cognition and orientation problems. You may feel like you are in a perpetual haze; performing simple tasks can be difficult, and your memory may be impaired. The good news is that you will not—or should not—be doing anything that requires concentration, such as driving. Appendix A lists several suggestions for promoting better sleep.

Weight loss. One of the outcomes of scoliosis surgery that many people welcome is a loss in weight. The rate of weight loss may shock you. I lost as much as two pounds *per day* for two weeks. Most people will taper off at a certain weight, then gradually regain some of it.

Incredible appetite—or none at all. After surgery, patients tend to fall into one of two extreme camps regarding appetite levels. Some patients feel perpetually famished, as I did. No matter how much I ate, I felt like I was starving. The medical explanation for this is that the body needs to take in a higher-than-usual number of calories to repair itself. But regardless of what and how much you eat, you will probably continue to lose weight for some time.

At the opposite extreme, some patients have little or no appetite whatsoever for weeks after surgery. This, too, has a medical explanation: the painkilling drugs most patients take postoperatively wreak havoc with your digestive system and can temporarily "disable" hunger. This loss of appetite can be exacerbated by the other problems many patients experience concurrently—pain, fatigue, and even stress and emotional anguish.

Whatever your level of appetite, it is important that you eat a well-balanced diet to provide your body with the nutrients it needs to heal. You also need calories as a source of energy to combat the weakness and fatigue you will almost certainly experience while recovering.

Constipation. Two things will cause constipation after surgery. First, in the hospital you will recall a point where your intestines began working again after having been shut down temporarily by anesthesia. After reaching that point, your digestive system still needs some time to begin producing and passing bowel movements. In addition, narcotic painkillers and iron supplements are extremely constipating.

There are many ways to combat constipation: over-the-counter laxatives and stool softeners, eating foods rich in fiber (such as fruit, bran, some cereals, and beans), drinking plenty of water or prune juice, consuming hot liquids (like coffee, tea, or soup), and even walking or other gentle exercise, which stimulates your digestive system. Weaning yourself off narcotics and iron supplements, if you are taking them, as soon as possible will obviously also assist with bowel regularity.

Menstrual problems. Most women get their period soon after the stress of surgery. Surgery may also cause irregular menstrual cycles for some time.

Other problems. In addition to the list of common problems listed above, the range of other complications people experience is extensive and sometimes downright strange. Doctors cannot always explain why people have such unusual problems. Personally, I had a strange experience with my sense of smell—things simply smelled wrong to me. For example, for three weeks after surgery, a perfume my mother wore inexplicably smelled like burnt toast. Since the way food tastes is largely a function of how it smells, I found many foods tasted "off"—not necessarily bad, just not what I expected them to taste like. As another example, many people have significant trouble maintaining body temperature; one minute they are freezing, the next they are burning up. Some patients report diminished hearing, or poorer eyesight. Again, be patient. Though confusing and frustrating, these kinds of problems are not unusual and will subside on their own.

Postoperative Pain Management

You will almost certainly need medication to control your pain after surgery. Because everyone *experiences* pain differently, and *responds* to drugs differently, the specific medication one takes, how often one takes it, and how long one takes it will vary from person to person. Your surgeon will prescribe a drug or recommend an over-the-counter medication that he or she feels will best meet your particular needs. However, only *you* can evaluate the success of that medication. Frequent modifications to the type, dosage, and frequency may be necessary.

The pain management drugs typically prescribed for scoliosis surgery fall into one of two camps: over-the-counter Tylenol (acetaminophen) in multiple forms, and prescription narcotics.

Tylenol (acetaminophen)

Tylenol, like most drugs available over-the-counter, is not as strong as prescription-strength painkillers. But for many individuals who have just had scoliosis surgery—especially younger patients—the pain relief provided by Tylenol is as good or almost as good as that provided by the stronger prescription medications. More importantly, Tylenol does not induce the myriad of side effects common to narcotics. Furthermore, Tylenol is inexpensive, especially if acetaminophen is purchased in a generic form.

If you are having trouble sleeping, you might want to try Tylenol PM. Tylenol PM combines acetaminophen with the same active ingredient as in Benadryl® (diphenhydramine hydrochloride), an antihistamine for allergies. This ingredient does nothing to reduce pain but does induce marked drowsiness in most people. If you are also suffering from allergies, this could be a good choice.

You may have found through your own experience with various over-the-counter analgesics to relieve minor aches and pains (like headaches) that Tylenol does not work as well for you as other drugs, such as Advil (ibuprofen), Aleve (naproxen), or plain aspirin. Everyone has his or her favorite over-the-counter painkiller. Unfortunately, as mentioned in Chapter 5, all of these common analgesics *except* Tylenol are in a class of drugs called nonsteroidal anti-inflammatory drugs (NSAIDs) that may interfere with the fusion process. NSAIDs can slow the rate at which your newly-fused spine solidifies or, worse, prevent it from fusing altogether. Doctors differ in their advice on how long you should wait after surgery before taking NSAIDs again. Some say six weeks, others two or three months. Fortunately, most people do not need painkillers continuously after the first month or so, so this may be a moot issue.

Acetaminophen is not without some risks, however. Large doses of acetaminophen can cause liver damage, as can smaller doses taken continuously for a long time. This effect is exacerbated if you consume three or more alcoholic drinks per day. Be sure to follow the drug manufacturer's guidelines for a safe dosage.

Narcotic Analgesics
The most commonly prescribed medications for postoperative pain management belong to a class of drugs called narcotic analgesics. These are also called *opioid* analgesics because the primary painkiller in these medications is derived from an opiate. In this context, the term "narcotic" simply means that the drug is potentially *habit-forming* (addictive); analgesic means "pain relieving." There are several types of narcotic analgesics. The most commonly prescribed drugs blend acetaminophen—the active ingredient in Tylenol—with a small amount of codeine or a chemically-related drug. The acetaminophen enhances the effect of the codeine.

There are four types of narcotic analgesics that combine codeine or a similar drug with acetaminophen. The most commonly prescribed is *hydrocodone*. A partial list of brand names include Anexsia®, Anolor, Bancap-HC,

Dolacet®, Lorcet®, Lortab®, Norco®, T-Gesic®, Vicodin®, and Zydone®. Other types you may be prescribed include *propoxyphene* (Darvocet®, Propacet®, Wygesic®), *oxycodone* (Endocet®, Percocet®, Roxicet®, Roxilox®, Tylox®), or *acetaminophen and codeine* (Capital® with Codeine Suspension, Phenaphen® with Codeine, Tylenol with Codeine).

These drugs vary in the exact amount of codeine (or equivalent) and acetaminophen in each dose. Many drugs have numbers after their name, such as "Lorcet 10/650." This means that this particular drug has 10 mg of the opiate (in this case, hydrocodone) mixed with 650 mg of acetaminophen. The higher the numbers, the stronger the medication. You may also see the name of the drug as "APAP," such as "Hydrocodone/APAP." APAP stands for *acetyl-p-aminophenol*, which is just the chemical name for acetaminophen.

Narcotic analgesics are powerful painkillers and have some significant side effects. Severe constipation, fatigue, and dizziness are the most common problems associated with taking these drugs. Mixing narcotics with certain other medications that also cause drowsiness, like cold and flu remedies and antidepressants, may result in a dangerous level of sedation. More importantly, some narcotics are habit-forming. The more you take them, the less powerful their effect will be because your body will develop a tolerance to them. Over time, you could find yourself needing to take progressively higher doses more frequently to get any effect at all. In addition, the high levels of acetaminophen in these drugs can cause liver damage, especially if you drink a lot of alcoholic beverages.

Because of the side effects and risks of these drugs, *your goal should be to wean yourself off narcotics as soon as possible.* As your pain begins to subside, take the narcotic less often and try to take over-the-counter Tylenol more frequently instead. I found during my recovery that my pain was worst first thing in the morning and at night. After a few days of taking only Vicodin several times a day, I switched to only taking Vicodin when I woke up and just before I went to sleep, and I took extra-strength Tylenol (500 mg capsules) during the day whenever my pain level increased. Vicodin made me drowsy so taking it at night helped me to sleep.

The maximum recommended dose of acetaminophen for an adult is 4000 mg per day. Be sure to track how much acetaminophen there is in the narcotic you are consuming, in addition to the amount of acetaminophen you are consuming in a pure form (such as Tylenol). I found that keeping a simple journal of all the medications I took—including date and time, name of the drug, and dosage—was useful to help me ensure that I was not taking too much of any medication, or taking it too often.

Of course, there are many ways to control your pain without taking drugs. These were discussed in Chapter 3. The most effective methods post-operatively include simple exercises (especially walking), stretching, and relaxation techniques. Chiropractic care, massage therapy, or any other pain management technique that places force on your back should not be pursued until your back is healed.

Diet and Nutrition

Few surgeons will put restrictions on what you can eat while recovering from surgery. While it is healing, your body will need more calories than normal. You will almost definitely lose weight, too, as your body turns to your fat stores to supplement the calories it takes in from the food you are eating. While you should not worry too much about what specific foods you eat, you should still try to eat relatively healthily and include foods from the five food groups: fruits, vegetables, breads, dairy products, and meat. Vegetarians may find the lack of meat in their diet to be problematic, and may need to obtain added protein from other food sources. The better you eat, the higher your energy levels will be and the faster you will heal.

You should also drink *plenty* of liquids. Drinking large amounts of liquids will help relieve the constipation that accompanies taking narcotic painkillers. Prune juice, in particular, has a known laxative effect. You should limit your intake of caffeinated beverages like coffee, tea, or soda because caffeine dehydrates your body. You can, of course, try decaffeinated versions of these drinks.

Almost every vitamin and mineral plays some role in helping your body heal. If you eat a well-balanced diet, you will probably get all the nutrients you need to help your body heal itself. Of course, few people eat an ideal diet no matter how hard they try. Taking a multi-vitamin, therefore, may be helpful. Unless your surgeon instructed you to continue taking iron supplements after surgery, be sure to get a multi-vitamin that does not contain iron. Iron supplements cause constipation, which you certainly want to avoid if you are also taking narcotics.

Taking Care of Your Incision Site and Scars

Your incision site and scar(s) need little maintenance. However, there are a few things worth knowing:

- Your incision will most likely have been closed with sutures (stitches) that will harmlessly dissolve into your body. If so, there will be nothing to remove postoperatively. Some surgeons prefer, and in some cases must, use surgical staples or non-dissolvable sutures, either of which will need to be removed at a later date. Removing staples and sutures is fairly quick and painless.

- An adult's incision will usually heal ("seal up") within two weeks. Children's incisions will typically heal faster. The healing process may take longer, however, for individuals with weak immune systems, those taking steroids for other medical conditions, or those with certain other disorders.

- The Steri-Strips applied over your incision will begin to fall off after two to three weeks. You should not pick at them during this time, but if they are still hanging on after three weeks, peel them off carefully.

- Some people experience intense postoperative itching around the incision site. This may be caused either by the healing wound or by the adhesive on the Steri-Strips. It is important that you do not scratch your incision. If the itching becomes unbearable, your doctor may be able to prescribe a cream to relieve this. The itchiness will diminish with time.

- Some surgeons recommend you keep a sterile dressing (bandage) over your incision site for the first week or two after surgery. If you have a dressing, be sure to keep it clean and dry, and change it whenever necessary.

- Your incision will be watertight by the time you leave the hospital. Even so, you should not completely submerge yourself in water (in a bath, hot tub, swimming pool, etc.) for the first month or so. This can cause the Steri-Strips to fall off prematurely and may increase your susceptibility to infection. Taking a shower is usually fine (check with your surgeon), but you should avoid spraying high-pressure water directly onto the incision.

- A small amount of bleeding or the discharge of a yellow fluid from the incision site for the first week or two is not abnormal and is not necessarily cause for alarm. Call your surgeon immediately if this discharge becomes excessive, continues for more than two weeks, or emits a foul odor (which could be a sign of infection).

- Your scar (or scars) will initially have a bright red appearance, be rough to the touch, and be raised above the skin. The redness is caused by numerous new blood vessels that form to nourish the tissues damaged during surgery. Scars in children typically become progressively redder for a few months, while in adults the level of redness may stay relatively constant. The intensity of coloration will begin to diminish three to twelve months after surgery. During this time, the scar will also begin to flatten and soften. The color will eventually be closer to white.

- Newly-formed scars are highly susceptible to sunburn and excessive sunlight may permanently "burn-in" some of the redness of the scar. You should avoid exposing your scar to sunlight for a few weeks after surgery.

- Though no research studies have proved this, some people claim that lotions rich in Vitamin E, aloe, or an onion extract (used in the popular over-the-counter scar care gel Mederma®) can reduce the harshness, inflammation, and redness of a scar. You should not apply any creams, lotions or gels to your scar until it is sufficiently healed (about three weeks after surgery).

Returning to Work or School

You should return to work or school whenever *you* decide that you are ready. No matter what, though, you should not plan on returning for *at least* three weeks after surgery. Most patients (especially older adults) will need more time than this.

The biggest challenge to resuming your work or school schedule will be fighting intermittent fatigue. Your energy levels will waiver for some time after surgery, and you may find it difficult to stay focused for continuous periods. This may not be a significant obstacle if, for example, you work for an employer who will let you go home early if you are not feeling well, or if you are in college and have only one or two classes per day. This is obviously much more of a problem if you have a job that requires a minimum number of hours per day, or if you are in school and have classes all day.

If you need to drive to work or school, you should be extremely careful if you are still taking narcotic painkillers. Narcotics cause drowsiness that can be dangerous while driving. This effect can last hours and is often unpredictable. For your own safety, try to find an alternate way to get to and from work or school.

A few suggestions:

Tell your employer or teachers about your condition. They may make concessions to help you recover. Often it is better to have you at work or school contributing less than usual rather than not to have you there at all. High school or younger students should get a note from their orthopedist or other doctor excusing them from physical education courses, sports, or other school activities that could jeopardize the healing fusion or that would completely exhaust the student.

If you have a desk job, get a comfortable chair. Your employer or your health insurance may cover this expense if prescribed by a doctor.

Carry supportive pillows with you. You may need to prop your head, neck, or back against something soft and flexible.

Get a second set of school books. You will not be able to carry a backpack on your shoulders for a while. If someone cannot carry it for you, consider obtaining a second set of books: leave one set in a locker at school and keep one set at home for homework and studying.

Get a home tutor if you need one. Some school districts can provide a tutor at little or no cost to you.

Sex While Recovering

Scoliosis surgery does not preclude you from having a normal sex life. If you are sexually active, use common sense in deciding when to resume having sex after surgery. For a short time after surgery you may be in too much pain to have sex, and pain and fatigue may diminish your sex drive. Your pain and alertness levels will fluctuate during the day, often in a predictable pattern. If you are aware of these patterns, you may be able to plan your sexual activity for times in the day when you feel your best.

Certain sexual positions may be uncomfortable given your inability to bend your back. Because thrusting may be difficult for a heterosexual man who has recently had surgery, it might be easier if the woman is on top during sex. A heterosexual woman recovering from surgery may also be more comfortable on top, because the weight of her partner on her body may be painful. Alternatively, both men and women may find a side-to-side position more comfortable. Homosexual couples will need to experiment to find comfortable sexual positions. In general, the partner who has had surgery should take the less active role during sex. Oral sex, manual sex, or masturbation may be less painful alternatives to intercourse.

If you have been instructed to wear a postoperative brace, you should wear it during sex if you will remain in an upright position. Note that the edges of the brace can hurt your partner.

Couples should practice a reliable means of birth control for at least six months after surgery. See *Scoliosis Surgery and Pregnancy* in Chapter 4 for more information.

Postoperative Depression and Fears

You can be your own worst enemy after surgery. While recovering from scoliosis surgery, many people go through bouts of depression and anxiety, and may develop seemingly irrational fears of simple things or activities. This may happen immediately following surgery or even weeks or months later.

The cyclical nature of your physical recovery may grind on your emotions. One day you will feel great, and the next day you may feel like you have had a major setback. Sometimes you feel like you will just never get better. Simple things like walking, reading, or taking a shower may seem like monumental, impossible challenges. Believe me, this will subside.

You may feel very vulnerable in regard to your back for a while. Crowded places scared me at first. I was terrified that someone would inadvertently bump into my back, which I believed would cause excruciating pain. I found out through my own experimentation that the kind of bump one receives from casually walking into another really does not hurt. I was also worried about someone innocently slapping me on my back as a greeting. Amazingly, the first time I went out after surgery with a large group of people, five people did just that. It stung a little bit, but the experience actually helped me realize just how strong my back really was. After all, I still had my good old spine, but now it was reinforced with steel.

As your back heals, you may experience a wide array of frequently-changing, strange physical sensations. Some of these sensations can cause great concern, though usually there is nothing to worry about. For some time after surgery, for instance, many patients get the periodic feeling that they have dislodged the hardware in their back. They may get out of bed too quickly one morning and feel a sharp pain that they then attribute to having broken a rod. This kind of sudden, caught-off-guard fear can be terrifying.

Two weeks after my surgery, I developed a piercing headache that narcotic painkillers could not dampen. I searched the Internet for any information about a connection between intense headaches and surgery. I found a story of a woman who suffered from postoperative headaches for months before she found that a rod in her back had broken and was compressing a nerve that was causing those headaches. I panicked and called my surgeon to see if this could somehow be what was happening to me; it seemed awfully coincidental that I developed the worst headache of my life shortly after surgery. My surgeon suspected it was unrelated and advised me to go the emergency room. Returning to the same hospital at which I had my surgery just two weeks prior was an eerie feeling. A CAT scan revealed that my headache was caused by severe sinus congestion due to seasonal allergies. Sure enough, decongestants and antihistamines eliminated the headaches. The experience made me realize how terrified I was, perhaps just subconsciously, of a failure in my surgery. I was so scared that I may have needed to go through another surgical procedure to repair the damage that I did not want to go to the emergency room for fear of what it might mean.

When you have feelings like this, talk to someone. People who have gone through the same surgery as you will probably offer you the best perspective on your situation, and you will trust them because of your shared experiences. Scoliosis support groups can also provide invaluable emotional support. Of course, family and friends can help, too. If you feel that your depression or fears are so powerful that they restrict your life, you may need to seek professional counseling.

Follow-Up With Your Surgeon

Most surgeons will ask that you return to their office for a postoperative evaluation four to six weeks after surgery, then at three or four months, six to eight months, and one year after surgery, and then once a year after that. At each of these visits, your spine will be x-rayed and your Cobb angle computed to see if your curvature is stable, improving, or worsening, and to verify that the hardware is intact. Your surgeon may also increase your range of allowed activities and, if you are still taking pain medication, modify the type or dosage.

Most patients will not experience any unusual problems that require contacting their surgeon outside of routine follow-up visits during the weeks following surgery. There are a few rare situations, however, in which you should contact your surgeon immediately:

- *Your incision site is opening, oozing, smells foul, is inflamed, or otherwise does not seem normal.* You have probably developed an infection, or your sutures need to be re-stitched.

- *You have severe, persistent pain in a specific area of your spine.* This could indicate that a piece of hardware has become dislodged.

- *Your pain medication is not effective.* If your pain is unbearable and the pain medication your surgeon prescribed is not alleviating it, your surgeon may be able to prescribe an alternate medication or modify your dosage.

- *Numbness, tingling, or weakness in your arms or legs.* This could be a sign of neurological damage. This is usually temporary and will disappear on its own. It could also be a side effect of pain control medication.

- *You lose bowel or bladder control*

- *You develop a fever that persists*

Victory

The amazing thing about scoliosis surgery is that it is an event that changes people, not just physically, but mentally and emotionally, as well. Immediately after surgery, when you feel terrible and can barely move, you will probably be questioning why you did it. As you begin to recover from the initial physical trauma of the surgery, however, you will probably begin to feel not just better, but like a different person. The process of learning how to do things that you may have once taken for granted—such as walking, sleeping, or getting out of a chair—will be agonizing at first, but most people grow emotionally stronger from the experience.

You may also begin to revel in your new body. You will be standing straighter and may even be taller. Pains that once affected you will probably diminish or be eliminated completely. Your rib hump, if you had one, will be flatter. Your entire body will be more balanced and natural-looking. Regardless of whether anyone notices these changes in you, *you* will notice them, and this will give you a welcome, lasting boost of confidence and pride. 80% of patients who have had scoliosis surgery are pleased with the results, despite all the temporary setbacks associated with it.

One thing that helped me recover emotionally was to gradually un-do many of the alterations I had made to my home in preparation for surgery and to "return to normal" the things I changed in my environment during the more challenging phases of my recovery. When you are physically ready, small steps like removing your raised toilet seat when you no longer need it, stashing away your prescription painkillers, removing the multitude of pillows that will have probably have accumulated throughout your house, and finally moving objects off your countertops down to the lower cupboards are all beneficial in helping you feel like you and your life are truly normal again. These small but significant changes are the ones that will give you your greatest sense of achievement and a realization of your own personal power.

If you choose to pursue scoliosis surgery, I wish you the best of luck!

And remember: you can do it.

APPENDIX A

Getting Your House and Life in Order

This section is meant as a checklist for the things you may want to do before surgery or might need while recovering. Depending on the nature of your particular surgery, how well you adapt and recover, and how many caregivers will be able to assist you, you may not need all of the things listed here. Items that virtually everyone will need, however, are noted. Note that your insurance may cover some of these items, or the hospital may provide them free of charge.

Reaching Things Around the House

Your house or apartment is probably arranged in such a way that assumes you can bend or stretch to reach things. For some time after surgery, however, this may prove difficult. This section contains some suggestions on reorganizing your house to make things more accessible and to make you more comfortable.

Move frequently-used items closer to your natural level of reach. For example, move pots and pans stored in under-counter cupboards to above-counter cupboards, or just place them on your countertop.

Get a step stool. You may find a step stool useful if you cannot move commonly-used items to an easily-accessible level, especially if you are not particularly tall.

A grab tool. These are essentially long sticks with tongs at one end that enable you to grab things off the floor or from above without bending. These cost approximately $25 and are available at most pharmacies. The hospital may provide one.

Make lamps easier to use. For example, if the on/off switch of your bedside lamp is difficult to reach without bending or stretching, attach the lamp to an extension cord with a switch that you can position closer to your bed. You might want to get a "clap lamp" that switches on and off by clapping your hands, or get a touch lamp that just requires a light touch to activate.

A Good Chair

You will want at least one chair that provides good support, keeps you relatively upright, and is easy to get in and out of. You may find that seats like highly-padded couches are too low to the ground or unsupportive. A few good options:

An electric lift recliner. These are ideal. Using a handheld remote control, you can raise and lower the chair to help you sit down and stand up without bending your back. They also recline electrically, thus providing a nice alternative to sleeping in your bed. These are expensive: expect to pay $600-$1,300. You might, however, be able to rent one from a medical supply store. If you intend to buy one, you should order it six weeks in advance; these are typically limited production items that need to be special-ordered. Insurance may cover the cost.

A hip chair. Hip chairs are essentially high chairs with low backs. Getting on and off the chair without bending your back is easy. Though much less expensive than electric lift recliners ($200-$400), these chairs are not as comfortable and do not recline.

An office chair. Many office chairs provide good support, have high backs, recline, and can raise and lower. Office chairs are relatively inexpensive ($50-$250 for most models) and are available in a tremendous variety of sizes, styles, and colors. If you choose an office chair that reclines, make sure it has a way to lock the recline feature so that you do not quickly fall back when you sit in it, which could hurt your spine. Also make sure to purchase a chair with arms. These will help stabilize you when getting in or out of the chair.

Take a regular chair you already own and pad it. Sometimes a couple of thin but supportive pillows can transform an uncomfortable chair into a good one. Many wooden kitchen table chairs, for example, have desirable qualities like high backs and a solid, stable base. But leaning against hard wood can be quite uncomfortable with a healing back. Some pillows may be sufficient to make it tolerable. Old-fashioned rocking chairs can work well, too, if padded sufficiently.

Sleeping

Everyone initially has trouble sleeping after surgery. It will be challenging to find a comfortable position that you can maintain for long enough to get a restful sleep. This section contains a few suggestions to help minimize the discomfort.

Get a good bed. Chapter 3 outlined some ideas on selecting a bed. A hospital bed may be a good option with its many adjustments. Some insurance companies will pay for this if your doctor prescribes it. You may be able to rent a hospital bed.

Raise your bed. If you do not already have one, buy a simple metal bed frame to get your bed off the floor (about $50).

Get lots of pillows. You will need extra pillows to prop your head up in bed and to raise various parts of your body off of your bed while sleeping. I recommend getting several firm, small- to medium-size pillows. Some patients recommend a body pillow or wedge pillow.

Keep warm. Regardless of the indoor temperature, many patients have trouble keeping warm while recovering from surgery. This is normal but quite uncomfortable. You may want to stock-up on blankets, or purchase an electric blanket (but note that heating pads can be dangerous if applied over your healing wound).

Getting Dressed

Dressing yourself without bending your back or being able to lift your arms can be quite a challenge. In general, you want to be sure that you have an adequate supply of clothing that can be put on and taken off with minimal effort. Some items you may want to have an on-hand include:

Button-up shirts and sweaters. Raising your arms over your head may be impossible initially.

Slip-on shoes or slippers. Laces are obviously difficult to tie without bending. Make sure that the soles of the shoes do not easily slip.

Loose-fitting, elastic-band sweatpants. Some patients swell around the hips after surgery. This is a must if you have to wear a brace after surgery.

Dressing stick. This long stick with a "hand" at the end helps you pull up your pants without bending over.

Sock aid. It is very difficult to put on your own socks if you cannot bend. A sock aid is essentially an extended grip that helps you pull your socks up. Someone else may be able to do this for you.

Long undershirt (if you must wear a postoperative brace). Buy several of these. 100% cotton is best.

Bathing

You will most likely need some degree of help the first few times you bathe. Some people will need to be held up in the shower. Others will only need help drying off, especially to dry their backs. Some things you may wish to purchase include:

No-rinse cleansers. Until you can take a shower, you can use washcloths, shampoos, and cleansers that do not require water. Even if someone else can wash you, you may have trouble bending over at a sink for rinsing. Some patients will be able to shower unattended on the day they return from the hospital.

Stability in the shower or bath. You may have trouble maintaining a solid footing for a while after surgery, and a slip in the shower or bath could be disastrous. A simple solution that will be adequate for most patients is a non-slip shower/bath mat. If you find maintaining your balance to be a serious problem, you might want to purchase a chair for your shower or bath, or install grab handles to the walls of your shower or bath.

Sponge with long handle. This will assist you in washing your back, though initially you will have trouble raising your arms to use this.

Razor tied or taped to a stick. This is excellent for women who want to shave their legs but are unable to do so due to limited movement. Alternatively, women may want to have their leg hair removed (with wax, laser, or by other means) prior to surgery to avoid this issue altogether.

Using the Toilet

Raised toilet seat. Getting on and off a toilet without bending your back is quite a challenge. To make this easier, you can purchase products that provide a seating platform several inches about the toilet. You should purchase one with arms for added stability. These typically cost $30-$100 and are available at medical supply stores, some pharmacies, and even some hardware stores. Your hospital may provide one for you; you should check before purchasing one. Insurance will generally cover this cost.

Re-locate the toilet paper dispenser in front of you. You may not be able to turn to your side to reach it.

Toilet tissue aid. Some people will not be able to reach far enough to wipe themselves.

Eating and Drinking

Bendable straws. These enable you to drink while laying down or sitting in a reclined position. They also limit the extent to which you need to raise your arms to bring a drink closer to your mouth.

Eating tray. You will occasionally need to eat in bed or in a chair. This will keep things cleaner.

Plastic drinking bottles. Your grip and your coordination will be diminished after surgery. Accidents will happen. It is better to drop plastic bottles than glass. And a plastic bottle with a built-in spout or straw, or with a cap, will prevent spills.

Think smaller and lighter. Buy, prepare, and store food in smaller-size containers or cookware, which are lighter and therefore easier to handle. Metals and plastics are much lighter than glassware or ceramics.

Stock up on prepared frozen and non-perishable foods that you can cook quickly and easily, or make your own foods and freeze them.

Grocery delivery services. A small number of supermarket chains will deliver food to your door that can be ordered by phone or over the Internet.

Collect the menus of your favorite local restaurants that deliver. Also check to see what food delivery services like Take-Out Taxi can supply.

Getting Around

A cane or walker. Most people will not need one, but older patients or those who have had a particularly extensive surgery may find walking without assistance difficult. You should not use a cane or walker without approval of your doctor and proper instruction on its use.

Handicapped placard for your vehicle. You can obtain a form for this from your Department of Motor Vehicles (or equivalent). It must be signed by a doctor. Even if you do not intend to drive until you can walk comfortably (good advice to follow), this placard could be hung in the vehicle of a caregiver or whomever may be driving you around to minimize your walk from the car.

Dial-a-ride programs. Most cities have transportation services for the disabled. You should consider yourself temporarily disabled. Some services are free, others are low-cost.

Medications

Tylenol or generic acetaminophen. It is best to buy a bottle of perhaps 100 tablets before surgery. You will almost certainly need them later. Be sure to buy the appropriate dosage size for your age.

Refill other prescription medications. If you take medications for a chronic condition, refill your prescriptions prior to surgery. Be sure to verify with your surgeon that taking these medications while recovering is okay.

Other Useful Items

Bell, buzzer, or other alert mechanism. You may need something to alert caregivers staying with you in your home that you need attention, especially at night when they may be sleeping. Baby monitors work well for this.

Hands-free telephone operation. Holding a phone up to your ear may be difficult. Speakerphones or headsets for your regular phone or cell phone may alleviate this problem.

APPENDIX B

Resources

Internet Sites

See the author's website, www.CurvedSpine.com, for a continuously updated list of good Internet sites on scoliosis.

National Scoliosis Organizations

Scoliosis Association, Inc.
P.O. Box 811705
Boca Raton, FL 33481-1705
Phone: (800) 800-0669
Fax: (561) 994-2455
www.scoliosis-assoc.org
scolioassn@aol.com

The Scoliosis Association, Inc. (SAI) is a nonprofit organization that provides information, help, and referrals to scoliosis patients, their families, and medical professionals through national support groups, information hotlines, and a publication called BACKTALK. The Association has available videos, books, special articles, fact sheets in English and Spanish, and other useful resources. In addition, SAI raises funds for scoliosis research and sponsors spine conferences in major cities that update and inform patients, families, and medical professionals about the current status, management, and treatment of scoliosis and related spinal conditions. Visit SAI's website for a national listing of local support groups.

National Scoliosis Foundation, Inc.
5 Cabot Place
Stoughton, MA 02072
Phone: (800) 673-6922
Fax: (781) 341-8333
www.scoliosis.org
nsf@scoliosis.org

The National Scoliosis Foundation (NSF) is a nonprofit organization that promotes public awareness and medical research about scoliosis. NSF provides education and support for patients and healthcare professionals through videos, books, brochures, local chapters, conferences, and postural screening training sessions. NSF can also help establish a scoliosis screening program for adolescents in your local schools. Full-time assistance is available Monday through Thursday, 9:00 a.m. to 4:30 p.m. EST, by calling 800-NSF-MYBACK (800-673-6922).

Scoliosis Research Society
611 East Wells Street
Milwaukee, WI 53202
Phone: (414) 289-9107
Fax: (414) 276-3349
www.srs.org

The Scoliosis Research Society (SRS) is primarily a professional organization for health care professionals who treat scoliosis, but it also serves as a *de facto* certification body for scoliosis surgeons. You should check with the SRS to verify that your preferred surgeon is a member; an updated listing of all SRS members is posted on their website. The website also contains graphics and x-ray examples to help explain scoliosis, as well as a glossary with some terms not defined in this book.

Other Books on Scoliosis

As mentioned in the Preface, this book is only applicable for those who are confronting scoliosis surgery. Topics such as the importance of early detection and bracing options for adolescents are not explored here. Three books nicely fill those gaps.

Brooke Lyons et al. *Scoliosis: Ascending the Curve.* New York: M. Evans and Company, 1999.

Co-authored with an orthopedic surgeon, a clinical psychologist, and a family therapist, *Ascending the Curve* takes a holistic perspective on diagnosing and treating scoliosis. Particular emphasis is given to the emotional aspects of coping with scoliosis. This book is especially good for adolescents because it has several inspiring stories of adolescents who have worn braces or undergone surgery. Ms. Lyons wrote this book while she was still in high school, so it easy for her to relate to the experiences and emotions of younger patients. Parents of adolescents with scoliosis will get a lot out of this book, too.

Neuwirth, Michael and Kevin Osborn. *The Scoliosis Sourcebook.* New York: Contemporary Books, 2001.

Written by an orthopedic surgeon together with a professional writer, this book provides fascinating insight into scoliosis from a surgeon's perspective. I recommend this book above the other two listed here for those who are confronting scoliosis surgery. For adolescents confronting bracing or for concerned parents, family members and friends who simply want to know more about scoliosis, either of the other two books is equally appropriate. *The Scoliosis Sourcebook* also contains an excellent chapter on degenerative scoliosis and addresses scoliosis caused by other conditions better than the other books. At times a bit technical, this is clearly a book for more advanced readers.

Schommer, Nancy. *Stopping Scoliosis: The Whole Family Guide to Diagnosis and Treatment*. New York: Avery, 2002.

Full of interviews with spine surgeons and replete with anecdotes from those who have worn back braces or undergone surgery, *Stopping Scoliosis* is a very readable, compassionate survey of diagnosing and treating scoliosis that is suitable for readers of all ages. This is the best book for those who want a fairly short, easy to read, solid overview of diagnosing and treating scoliosis. Either of the other two books mentioned in this section is more detailed, but at the expense of being longer and more technical. *Stopping Scoliosis* provides most of its information through interview transcripts and personal stories, a format that some people may prefer but others may find less accessible.

Glossary

Adolescent scoliosis A lateral spinal curvature that appears before the on-set of puberty and before an individual is skeletally mature

AIS Adolescent Idiopathic Scoliosis

allograft Bone for spine grafting taken from a human cadaver

anterior The front, or from the front. The opposite is *posterior* (back, or from the back).

A/P Anterior/posterior, in the context of (1) an A/P x-ray, which is taken with the patient facing the x-ray machine, or (2) scoliosis surgery in which incisions are made both from the front (anterior) and from the back (posterior).

apex The most deviated vertebra in a scoliotic spine; the "peak" of a curve. There may be more than one apex if there are multiple curves.

autologous In the context of donating blood, this means donating your own blood for use during your surgery

autogenous see *autograft*

autograft Bone for grafting material taken from your ribs or pelvis that will be used during your surgery

bending films/x-rays X-rays of your back taken while you are laying down and bending your torso as hard as you can to the right or left. These indicate how flexible your spine is and can be used to predict how much correction scoliosis surgery may achieve in your case.

BMP Bone Morphogenetic Protein, a natural material used to augment bone grafts. BMP may increase the likelihood of a successful fusion and can accelerate the rate at which the fusion process takes place.

cervical The section of spine in the neck, above the thoracic section. The cervical section of the spine comprises seven vertebrae.

Cobb method or Cobb angle The name of the method by which the severity of a scoliotic curve is measured (*the Cobb Method*). The resulting degree measurement is called the *Cobb angle*.

coccyx The lowest part of the spine, also called the tailbone

compensation In the context of scoliosis surgery, an individual is said to be *compensated* when his or her head is centered above the pelvis. The opposite of *decompensation*.

compensatory curve A secondary curve (there are sometimes two) that develops in order to help maintain normal body alignment (compensation)

concave The inside of a curve. Concave is the opposite of convex.

congenital scoliosis Scoliosis caused by a condition (typically, malformed vertebrae) with which one was born

contraindicated Not appropriate for—the opposite of *indicated*

convex The outside of a curve (the opposite of concave). A curve that bends to the right (from the perspective of the person with scoliosis) is said to have *right convexity*.

crankshaft effect A phenomenon that may affect individuals who have scoliosis surgery before reaching skeletal maturity in which the front (anterior) portion of the spine continues to grow and deform while the rear (posterior) portion remains held in place. This leads to a unique spinal deformation.

DBM Demineralized Bone Matrix, a variant of traditional allograft bone that uses extracted proteins taken from a human cadaver to enhance fusion

decompensation A potential outcome of scoliosis surgery in which the spine becomes imbalanced such that the head is not centered over the pelvis

discectomy The surgical removal of all or part of one or more intervertebral discs. Also spelled *diskectomy*.

discs, intervertebral Rings of cartilage surrounding a spongy core that separate two vertebrae and cushion impacts to the spine

double major curve Also called an "S" curve, this refers to a scoliotic spine with two major (structural) curves

endoscopic A surgical method in which an endoscope—an instrument with a tiny video camera inside it—is used to visually explore the chest cavity. Also called *thoracoscopic*.

facet joints The bony parts of a vertebra that connect it to other vertebrae

flatback A condition in which the normal lordosis (inward curve) of the lower back is lost and the lower back instead appears flat

Foley catheter The name of the tube inserted into one's urethra to drain urine after surgery

fusion The surgical process of transforming two or more adjacent vertebrae into one solid, continuous piece of bone

graft Fragments of bone taken from one's own body or from a cadaver and placed at the spinal fusion site to promote the fusion process

Harrington rod The name of the first instrument (rods) used in scoliosis surgery to stabilize a scoliotic curve

hemothorax A surgical complication involving the inadvertent drainage of blood into the lungs

idiopathic Unknown origin or cause

indicated Appropriate for (in the context of a particular medicine or procedure)

instrumentation Hardware (rods, screws, hooks, etc.) used to straighten and hold a scoliotic curve

IV Acronym for intravenous. An "IV" is a system that continuously delivers medicines, blood, or other fluids into your body through a needle inserted into a vein.

kyphosis This word has two somewhat conflicting meanings. It means both the normal curve of the upper back *and* it is sometimes used to describe an excess curvature (a condition commonly called hunchback or roundback). The implied meaning is usually clear in context. For example, a surgeon might say that he "can surgically restore normal kyphosis," or that one has "moderate scoliosis with just mild kyphosis."

lateral Side-to-side. A scoliotic spine has a lateral curvature as opposed to a front-to-back curvature (though an individual with scoliosis may also have the latter).

level(s) A number of vertebrae. Usually used in the context of discussing how many vertebrae will be fused or instrumented ("We need to fuse five levels"). Also called *segment(s)*.

logrolling A procedure used in hospitals while a patient is recovering in bed to turn the patient on either of his or her sides without bending or twisting the back. This is done by placing a sheet under the patient and then having one or two nurses carefully pull up one side of the sheet to roll the patient to the other side.

lordosis This word has two somewhat conflicting meanings. It means both the normal inward curve of the lower back *and* it is sometimes used to describe the absence of that normal curve (a condition commonly called flat back). The implied meaning is usually clear in context.

lumbar The lowest region of the spine, comprising five vertebrae. Above the lumbar region is the thoracic region, and below it is the sacrum.

midline A conceptual vertical line that indicates the true left-right midpoint of the spine

morselized bone Ground-up bone fragments used as grafts to promote fusion

narcotic analgesic A class of strong painkilling medications that may be addictive

nonstructural curve A curvature that is not fixed, or rigid. Often called a compensatory, secondary, or minor curve.

nonstructural scoliosis A generally mild, temporary case of scoliosis caused by poor posture, injury, or illness

NSAID Non-steroidal anti-inflammatory drug. Most commonly, these are known as over-the-counter painkillers like Advil, Aleve, and aspirin. Compared to narcotics, these are less powerful and have fewer side effects. Tylenol (acetaminophen) is *not* an anti-inflammatory drug and is not in this class. Some NSAIDs require a prescription.

orthopedics The branch of medicine that deals with disorders of the skeletal system

orthopedist Synonym for orthopedic surgeon

osteotomy The separation of a fused portion of spine into distinct segments that approximate vertebrae. Essentially the reverse of spinal fusion.

P/A Posterior/anterior, usually in the context of a P/A x-ray, which is taken with the patient facing away from the x-ray machine

PCA Patient Controlled Analgesia. A PCA is a machine that administers a continuous dosage of painkilling medication intravenously to a patient and also allows the patient to augment the continuous dosage with extra bursts of medication as needed.

pedicle The part of a vertebra that connects the rear (posterior) elements of the vertebra to the anterior (front) of the vertebra, which is also called the vertebral body. Pedicle screws would be placed in this section of bone.

pleura The outer lining of the lung

pneumothorax A possible surgical complication of scoliosis surgery, a pneumothorax is air temporarily trapped between the lung and chest wall.

posterior The back, or from the back (rear). The opposite of anterior.

pseudarthrosis The failure of some or all of the vertebrae involved in a fusion to fuse successfully. Also spelled *pseudoarthrosis*.

resection The cutting away of a section of bone, such as one or more ribs as part of a thoracoplasty

rib hump The cosmetic deformity of ribs that results from the rotation of a scoliotic spine in the thoracic region. The rotation forces some ribs to curve outward, thereby creating a hump on an individual's back that is most visible when the individual bends forward.

rotation The twisting of a spine around its vertical axis. Most scoliotic spines have some degree of rotation in addition to a lateral (side-to-side) curvature.

sacrum A large section of bone at the bottom of the spine between the bottom-most lumbar vertebra (L5) and the coccyx (tailbone). In developing infants, the sacrum is actually five distinct vertebrae; these vertebrae fuse together as one grows. The sacrum is sometimes denoted S1.

sagittal curves The front-to-back curves of a normal spine in the upper back (kyphosis) and lower back (lordosis). One goal of scoliosis surgery is to restore these natural curves, though not all individuals with scoliosis have abnormal sagittal curves.

segmental instrumentation Used in almost every scoliosis surgery performed today, segmental instrumentation (screws and hooks) can be attached to rods at multiple vertebrae, or segments, to achieve optimal correction of the curve.

selective fusion A fusion and instrumentation of only the structurally-curved sections of a spine; the compensatory curves are not fused or instrumented in the hope that they will correct on their own once the structural curve is corrected.

skeletal maturity A person's body is "skeletally mature" when his or her bones are no longer growing. This usually occurs when a female is 14-16 or a male is around 16-18 years old. Skeletal maturity is determined by measuring the amount of bone that has formed on the upper edge of the pelvis, an indication called the *Risser sign*.

structural curve   Also called a primary curve, this is the "true" scoliotic curve. In contrast, a compensatory curve is a curve that is merely curving in reaction to the structural curve.

structural scoliosis   Scoliosis caused by a presumably genetic or known medical condition

thoracic   The section of spine in the middle back, between the cervical (neck) and lumbar (lower back) sections. The thoracic section of the spine comprises twelve vertebrae (T1-T12) and supports the rib cage.

thoracolumbar curve   A structural curvature that spans both the thoracic and lumbar regions of the spine

thoracoplasty   A surgical procedure to reduce the rib hump often associated with thoracic curves by removing sections of one or more protruding ribs

thoracoscopic surgery   A minimally-invasive surgical technique in which the spine is accessed through tiny incisions into which an *endoscope* is inserted

TLSO   Thoracic lumbar sacral orthoses. A fiberglass brace that some patients must wear for several months after scoliosis surgery.

vertebrae   The twenty-four bones that, together with the sacrum and coccyx, comprise the spine

Works Cited

[1] An HS, Simpson JM, Glover JM, Stephany J. *Comparison between allograft plus demineralized bone matrix versus autograft in anterior cervical fusion. A prospective multi-center study.* Spine 1995; 20: 2211-16.

[2] Brown CW, Orme TJ, Richardson HD. *The rate of pseudarthrosis (surgical non-union) in patients who are smokers and patients who are nonsmokers: a comparison study.* Spine 1986; 9: 942-3.

[3] Thalgott JS, Cotler HB, Sasso RC, LaRocca H, Gardner V. *Postoperative infections in spinal implants. Classification and analysis -- a multicenter study.* Spine 1991: 8: 981-4.

[4] Betz, RR, et al. *Comparison of anterior and posterior instrumentation for correction of adolescent thoracic idiopathic scoliosis.* Spine 1999 Feb 1;24(3):225-39

[5] Picetti GD, Pang D, Bueff HU. *Thoracoscopic techniques for the treatment of scoliosis: early results in procedure development.* Neurosurgery 2002 Oct; 51(4):978-84

[6] Betz, RR, et al. *Thoracoscopic anterior instrumentation.* See http://www.spineuniverse.com/displayarticle.php/article498.html

[7] Heary, RF, et al. *Persistent iliac crest donor site pain: independent outcome assessment.* Neurosurgery 2002 Mar;50(3):510-6

[8] Burger EL, Baratta RV, King AG, Easton R, Lu Y, Solomonow M, Riemer BL. *The memory properties of cold-worked titanium rods in scoliosis constructs.* Spine 2005 Feb 15;30(4):375-9.

[9] Kim YJ, Bridwell KH, Lenke LG, Rinella AS, Edward C 2nd. *Pseudarthrosis in primary fusions for adult idiopathic scoliosis: incidence, risk factors, and outcome analysis.* Spine. 2005 Feb 15;30(4):468-74.

[10] Lantz CA, Chen J. *Effect of chiropractic intervention on small scoliotic curves in younger subjects: a time-series cohort design.* J Manipulative Physiol Ther (United States), Jul-Aug 2001, 24(6) p385-93

Index

About the Author

David Wolpert wrote the first edition of *Scoliosis Surgery: The Definitive Patient's Reference* in 2003 while recovering from scoliosis surgery. David's experience with scoliosis dates back to his teenage years, when he wore a Milwaukee Brace. His curve continued to progress into adulthood, ultimately requiring surgery in December, 2002. David had an excellent surgical outcome.

David also is the co-author of *The Human Fabric: Unleashing the Power of Core Energy in Everyone* (Aviri Publishing, 2004). Visit www.theHumanFabric.com to learn more about this title.

When not writing or helping scoliosis patients, David is a software product marketing manager. David has over ten years of diverse experience working with technology companies in a variety of technical and business roles.

David holds a B.S. in History from Carnegie Mellon University and an MBA from the University of Texas. A native of Detroit, today David resides in Austin.

Notes

Notes

Notes

Notes

Order a Copy of this Book

This title is not available in bookstores. Additional copies can be ordered from:

- Amazon.com

- The National Scoliosis Foundation — (800) 673-6922, or online at www.scoliosis.org

- The Scoliosis Association, Inc. — (800) 800-0669, or online at www.scoliosis-assoc.org

Medical professionals, librarians, and international customers interested in this book should visit:

www.CurvedSpine.com/order

or fax an inquiry to: (484) 492-7299